COMPREHENSIVE GUIDELINES FOR THYROID DISORDER MANAGEMENT

Innovative Approaches for Optimal Patient Outcomes

Dr. Yoshiki Kiyomizu

Copyright © 2024 by Dr. Yoshiki Kiyomizu

All rights reserved. No part of this book may be reproduced or transmitted in any form or by any means, electronic or mechanical, including photocopying, recording, or any information storage and retrieval system, without the prior written permission of the publisher, except for the use of brief quotations in a book review.

Preface

Thyroid disorders encompass a wide range of conditions that can significantly impact patient health and quality of life. From the subtle fluctuations of thyroid function to the more severe manifestations of thyroid disease, the complexity of these disorders requires a comprehensive approach to diagnosis, management, and treatment. It is with this understanding that we present "COMPREHENSIVE GUIDELINES FOR THYROID DISORDER MANAGEMENT: Innovative Approaches for Optimal Patient Outcomes."

The primary aim of this book is to provide a thorough and practical guide for healthcare professionals engaged in the management of thyroid disorders. This text is designed to bridge the gap between theoretical knowledge and clinical practice, offering evidence-based recommendations tailored to current standards and innovative approaches.

Structure and Content

The book is meticulously organized into several chapters, each addressing critical aspects of thyroid disorder management:

1. Thyroid Disorders: Overview - This introductory chapter provides a broad understanding of thyroid disorders, including their classification, epidemiology, and impact on health.

2. Diagnosis of Hyperthyroidism - Detailed insights into the diagnostic processes for hyperthyroidism, including biochemical evaluation, diagnostic testing, and management strategies.

3. Subclinical Hyperthyroidism - A focused discussion on the definition, prevalence, clinical

significance, and management of subclinical hyperthyroidism.

4. Thyroid Nodules/Goitre - An examination of the prevalence, evaluation methods, and management strategies for thyroid nodules and goitre.

5. Thyroid Emergencies and Perioperative Management - Covers critical emergencies like thyroid storm and myxoedema coma, alongside perioperative considerations for thyroid disease management.

6. Thyroiditis – Subacute and Acute Thyroiditis - Provides an in-depth analysis of subacute and acute thyroiditis, including diagnostic and treatment approaches.

7. Thyroid Cancer Management - Detailed guidelines on the management of thyroid cancer, from initial diagnosis to treatment and follow-up.

8. Postpartum Thyroiditis - A comprehensive review of postpartum thyroiditis, including its differentiation from Graves' disease, management, and implications for thyroid dysfunction in children and adolescents.

9. Graves' Ophthalmopathy - Discusses the incidence, definition, assessment, and treatment of Graves' ophthalmopathy, including innovative and evidence-based therapeutic approaches.

10. Implementation of Clinical Practice Guidelines (CPG) - Focuses on the practical aspects of implementing clinical practice guidelines for thyroid disorders, addressing facilitating and limiting factors, resource implications, and quality management indicators.

Purpose and Audience

This book is intended for clinicians, endocrinologists, family practitioners, and medical students who seek a comprehensive understanding of thyroid disorders and their management. The guidelines and recommendations presented are grounded in the latest research and clinical evidence, aiming to support practitioners in delivering optimal patient care.

In preparing this guide, I have drawn upon a wealth of clinical experience and recent advances in thyroid disorder management. It is my hope that this book will serve as a valuable resource, enhancing the knowledge and skills of healthcare providers and ultimately contributing to improved patient outcomes.

Conclusion

With this book, I invite you to explore and implement these comprehensive guidelines, fostering innovative approaches and striving for excellence in thyroid disorder management. Together, we can advance the standard of care and achieve optimal outcomes for our patients.

Dr. Yoshiki Kiyomizu
Clinical Researcher, Keio University Hospital, Tokyo, Japan

Acknowledgements

I extend my deepest gratitude to the numerous colleagues, researchers, and healthcare professionals who have contributed to the development of this work. Their insights and expertise have been invaluable in shaping the guidelines presented herein.

About the Author

Dr. Yoshiki Kiyomizu

Dr. Yoshiki Kiyomizu, born in Tokyo, Japan, is an esteemed Clinical Researcher at Keio University Hospital. He completed his entire academic journey at Tokyo University, earning his medical degree and specializing in endocrinology with a focus on thyroid disorder management. Dr. Kiyomizu's research is dedicated to advancing understanding and treatment of thyroid diseases, including hyperthyroidism, hypothyroidism, and thyroid cancer. His work contributes significantly to improving patient outcomes and developing innovative therapies in the field of thyroidology.

Abbreviations

1. ATD: Antithyroid Drug
   - Significance: Medications used to manage hyperthyroidism by inhibiting thyroid hormone synthesis.

2. CAS: Clinical Activity Score
   - Significance: A tool used to assess the severity and activity of Graves' Ophthalmopathy (GO).

3. DON: Dysthyroid Optic Neuropathy
   - Significance: A severe form of GO that can threaten vision due to compression of the optic nerve.

4. ECG/EKG: Electrocardiogram
   - Significance: A diagnostic tool used to assess heart function and can be affected by thyroid disorders.

5. FT4: Free Thyroxine

- Significance: A key thyroid hormone measured to assess thyroid function and diagnose disorders.

6. GO: Graves' Ophthalmopathy
   - Significance: An autoimmune condition affecting the eyes, often associated with Graves' disease.

7. GC: Glucocorticoid
   - Significance: Steroid hormones used in the treatment of inflammation and autoimmune conditions, including GO.

8. MRI: Magnetic Resonance Imaging
   - Significance: An imaging modality used to evaluate thyroid gland abnormalities and orbital changes.

9. RAI: Radioactive Iodine
   - Significance: A treatment for hyperthyroidism that can affect thyroid function and potentially exacerbate GO.

10. T3: Triiodothyronine
   - Significance: A thyroid hormone important for regulating metabolism, often measured in thyroid function tests.

11. T4: Thyroxine
   - Significance: The primary thyroid hormone, critical for metabolic regulation and assessed in thyroid function tests.

12. TSH: Thyroid-Stimulating Hormone
   - Significance: A pituitary hormone that regulates thyroid function; elevated or low levels indicate thyroid dysfunction.

13. TSHR: Thyroid-Stimulating Hormone Receptor
   - Significance: Receptor involved in thyroid hormone regulation and targeted by antibodies in autoimmune thyroid diseases.

14. TSAb: Thyroid-Stimulating Antibodies

- Significance: Antibodies that stimulate the thyroid gland, commonly associated with Graves' disease.

15. TT4: Total Thyroxine
   - Significance: Measures both bound and free thyroxine levels, providing a comprehensive view of thyroid function.

16. US: Ultrasound
   - Significance: An imaging technique used to evaluate thyroid nodules and gland morphology.

Table of Contents

Preface
- Introduction to the Book
- Purpose and Scope
- Acknowledgements
- Abbreviations
- Table of contents

Chapter 1: Thyroid Disorders: Overview
- Classification and Epidemiology
- Clinical Significance
- Impact on Health

Chapter 2: Diagnosis of Hyperthyroidism
- Biochemical Evaluation
- Diagnostic Testing
- Management Strategies

Chapter 3: Subclinical Hyperthyroidism
- Definition and Prevalence
- Clinical Significance
- Associated Risks

- Management

Chapter 4: Thyroid Nodules/Goitre
- Prevalence and Clinical Presentation
- Clinical Evaluation
- Diagnostic Imaging
- Fine Needle Aspiration Biopsy
- Molecular Testing
- Management Strategies

Chapter 5: Thyroid Emergencies and Perioperative Management
- Thyroid Storm
- Myxoedema Coma
- Perioperative Management

Chapter 6: Thyroiditis – Subacute and Acute Thyroiditis
- Subacute Thyroiditis (De Quervain's Thyroiditis)
- Diagnosis and Management
- Acute (Suppurative) Thyroiditis
- Treatment Approaches

Chapter 7: Thyroid Cancer Management
- Diagnostic Approaches
- Treatment Strategies
- Follow-Up and Surveillance

Chapter 8: Postpartum Thyroiditis
- Definition and Natural History
- Differentiation from Graves' Disease
- Management and Monitoring
- Thyroid Dysfunction in Children and Adolescents
- Conditions like Hashimoto's Thyroiditis
- Specific Syndromes (Turner Syndrome, Down Syndrome)

Chapter 9: Graves' Ophthalmopathy
- Overview and Incidence
- First-Line Treatment: High-Dose Intravenous Glucocorticoids
- Second-Line Treatment: Orbital Radiotherapy and Cyclosporine
- Rituximab and Other Emerging Therapies
- Management of Sight-Threatening GO

- Treatment for Moderate-to-Severe and Inactive GO
- Radioactive Iodine Therapy and Prophylaxis

Chapter 10: Implementation of Clinical Practice Guidelines (CPG)
- Facilitating and Limiting Factors
- Resource Implications
- Proposed Clinical Audit Indicators
- Quality Management Strategies

Key recommendations
Glossary
References

Chapter One
Thyroid Disorders: Overview

Thyroid disorders encompass a wide spectrum of diseases that result from abnormalities in the thyroid gland, which is a crucial part of the endocrine system. Located at the base of the neck, the thyroid gland regulates various metabolic processes in the body through the secretion of thyroid hormones, primarily thyroxine (T4) and triiodothyronine (T3). Disruptions in the function of the thyroid gland can lead to a variety of clinical conditions, primarily categorized into hypothyroidism, thyroid nodules, and thyroid cancer. Proper management of thyroid disorders is essential due to their far-reaching impact on various organ systems, as well as their prevalence in the general population.

Epidemiology of Thyroid Disorders

Thyroid disorders represent some of the most common endocrine diseases globally, affecting millions of individuals each year. The prevalence and incidence of these disorders vary based on geography, age, gender, and underlying etiological factors. Understanding the epidemiology of thyroid disorders is crucial for public health planning, screening, and prevention efforts.

Global Prevalence

The global burden of thyroid disease is significant, with estimates suggesting that approximately 200 million people worldwide are affected by some form of thyroid disorder. The prevalence of thyroid disorders is notably higher in regions where iodine deficiency is endemic, particularly in developing countries. Iodine deficiency remains the most preventable cause of thyroid dysfunction globally, despite the widespread implementation of iodization programs. In iodine-sufficient regions, autoimmune conditions, particularly

Hashimoto's thyroiditis and Graves' disease, are the leading causes of thyroid disorders.

Gender Disparities

Thyroid disorders are known to have a marked gender disparity, with women being disproportionately affected. It is estimated that women are five to ten times more likely to develop thyroid disorders compared to men. This increased susceptibility in women is often attributed to hormonal fluctuations, particularly during pregnancy, postpartum periods, and menopause, which can trigger or exacerbate thyroid dysfunction. Autoimmune thyroid disease, such as Hashimoto's thyroiditis, is also more common in women, with a prevalence rate of about 5-10% in females compared to 1-2% in males.

Age-Related Trends

The incidence of thyroid disorders also varies with age. While thyroid dysfunction can occur at any age, it is more common in older adults. Hypothyroidism, in particular, tends to increase in prevalence with advancing age, with a significant proportion of older adults being affected by subclinical or overt hypothyroidism. On the other hand, hyperthyroidism, particularly Graves' disease, often presents in younger adults, but toxic multinodular goiter and toxic adenoma are more commonly observed in older populations.

Regional Variations

Epidemiological studies have shown significant regional variations in the prevalence of thyroid disorders, largely driven by iodine status. In areas of iodine deficiency, endemic goiter and hypothyroidism are common, whereas in iodine-replete areas, autoimmune thyroid diseases such as Hashimoto's thyroiditis and Graves' disease predominate. For example, in South Asia and Sub-Saharan Africa, where iodine deficiency is still prevalent, the incidence of goiter and hypothyroidism remains high.

Conversely, in North America and Western Europe, where iodine sufficiency has been largely achieved, autoimmune thyroid disorders are the primary concern.

Impact of Lifestyle and Environmental Factors

Lifestyle and environmental factors also play a significant role in the epidemiology of thyroid disorders. Exposure to radiation, particularly in childhood, has been strongly linked to an increased risk of thyroid cancer and other thyroid dysfunctions. Dietary factors, including excessive iodine intake, selenium deficiency, and the consumption of goitrogens (substances that disrupt thyroid function), can influence thyroid health. Additionally, smoking has been associated with an increased risk of Graves' disease and a more severe course of ophthalmopathy in affected individuals.

Thyroid Cancer Epidemiology

Thyroid cancer, although less common than benign thyroid disorders, has been rising in incidence worldwide, particularly in high-income countries. This increase is partly attributed to enhanced detection through the widespread use of diagnostic imaging, such as ultrasound, which can identify small, asymptomatic thyroid nodules. Papillary thyroid carcinoma (PTC) is the most common type of thyroid cancer, accounting for approximately 80-85% of all cases. The prognosis for thyroid cancer is generally favorable, with a five-year survival rate exceeding 90% for most patients.

Thyroid Disorders in Special Populations

Certain populations are at increased risk for thyroid disorders, including pregnant women, neonates, and individuals with a family history of thyroid disease. During pregnancy, the demand for thyroid hormones increases significantly, and inadequate thyroid function can lead to complications such as preterm birth, preeclampsia, and neurodevelopmental deficits in the offspring. Neonatal thyroid screening is critical in detecting congenital hypothyroidism, which, if left untreated, can result in intellectual disability and growth failure.

In conclusion, thyroid disorders are prevalent worldwide and demonstrate significant variation based on factors such as geography, age, gender, and environmental exposures. Understanding these epidemiological trends is essential for improving diagnosis, treatment, and prevention strategies, ultimately leading to better patient outcomes.

Activation of Thyroid Hormone Synthesis and Secretion Leading to Excessive Hormone Release

Graves' disease is the predominant cause of primary hyperthyroidism, with prevalence rates ranging from 70% to 84% in various regions. This condition arises from the presence of anti-TSH receptor antibodies and has been linked to Yersinia infection. Other primary causes of hyperthyroidism include toxic adenoma and toxic multinodular goiter. Genetic studies on resected nodules have identified mutations in the TSH receptor gene, which result in the basal activation of the protein kinase A pathway, leading to increased T4 production and cell proliferation. This mutation also enhances the TSH receptor's affinity for TSH, further elevating thyroid hormone synthesis. Not all hot nodules are benign, and some may be malignant. Literature suggests that approximately 3.1% of hot nodules are diagnosed as thyroid cancer. Thyroid papillary carcinoma can also induce hyperthyroidism. Graves' disease may coexist with toxic adenoma, a condition known as Marine–Lenhart syndrome. Additionally, a rare group of patients may have diffuse non-autoimmune hyperthyroidism due to genetic mutations causing thyroid hormone production independent of TSH.

A. Excessive Release of Preformed Thyroid Hormones Due to Various Insults

The release of excessive thyroid hormones can occur due to the destruction of thyroid follicle cells, resulting in hyperthyroidism. This destruction may be caused by autoimmune conditions such as Hashimoto's thyroiditis, infections like subacute thyroiditis (viral) or Mycobacterium tuberculosis, cellulitis of the anterior neck, or physical trauma from rapidly growing anaplastic thyroid carcinoma or primary thyroid lymphoma.

B. Exposure to Extrathyroidal Sources of Thyroid Hormone

Thyroid hormones can also be sourced from extrathyroidal origins, either endogenous or exogenous. Endogenous sources include struma , a teratoma in the ovaries primarily composed of thyroid tissue, and metastatic thyroid carcinoma that secretes thyroid hormones. These cases are rare, with fewer than 100 reported since 1946. Exogenous sources, including over-the-counter thyroid supplements containing T3 or T4, are becoming increasingly common. These supplements are available online, are inexpensive, do not require a prescription, and offer privacy for individuals managing their own health.

C. Exogenous Sources of Thyroid Hormones

Exogenous thyroid hormones can be found in over-the-counter supplements that may not disclose their exact ingredients. Additionally, thyroid hormones can be ingested through animal thyroid glands, as evidenced by an outbreak of thyrotoxicosis linked to consumption of beef hamburgers containing thyroid hormone.

D. Excessive Thyroid Stimulation by Trophic Factors

Excessive stimulation of the thyroid gland can occur due to trophic factors such as thyroid-stimulating hormone (TSH) and other agents. TSHoma, a rare pituitary adenoma that secretes excess TSH and causes secondary hyperthyroidism, is one such condition. Similarly, gestational trophoblastic disease, which secretes β-HCG with partial structural similarity to TSH, can induce thyrotoxicosis. This condition is infrequent, affecting 2.0 per 1000 pregnancies, with only 7% showing biochemical thyrotoxicosis. Furthermore, iodine-rich contrast agents used in CT scans and angiographic procedures, as well as amiodarone used for tachyarrhythmias, can contribute to Jod-Basedow thyrotoxicosis due to the excess iodine. The prevalence of contrast-induced subclinical hyperthyroidism can be up to 2.66%, while hyperthyroidism may occur in up to 1.7% of cases. Amiodarone-induced thyrotoxicosis has a higher prevalence, ranging from 3.0% to 20.8%. Rare cases of thyrotoxicosis have also been reported with L-asparaginase chemotherapy, which causes transient thyrotoxicosis.

Chapter Two
Diagnosis of Hyperthyroidism

Biochemical Evaluation

The initial screening test for hyperthyroidism is the serum TSH measurement, which offers high sensitivity and specificity. To enhance diagnostic accuracy, both serum TSH and free T4 (fT4) levels should be evaluated. If fT4 levels are normal but TSH is suppressed, measuring free T3 (fT3) is recommended. In overt hyperthyroidism, both serum fT4 and fT3 are typically elevated, and serum TSH is usually suppressed to levels below 0.01 mIU/L.

Diagnostic Testing for Etiology

When expertise is available and Graves' disease is not evident from clinical history, thyroid ultrasound, including conventional grayscale and color flow Doppler, is recommended to investigate hyperthyroidism. Thyroid vascularity and peak systolic velocity (PSV) of the inferior thyroid artery are useful in differentiating between Graves' disease and thyroiditis, especially during pregnancy.

Figure 2-1: Diagnostic Algorithm for Suspected Hyperthyroidism

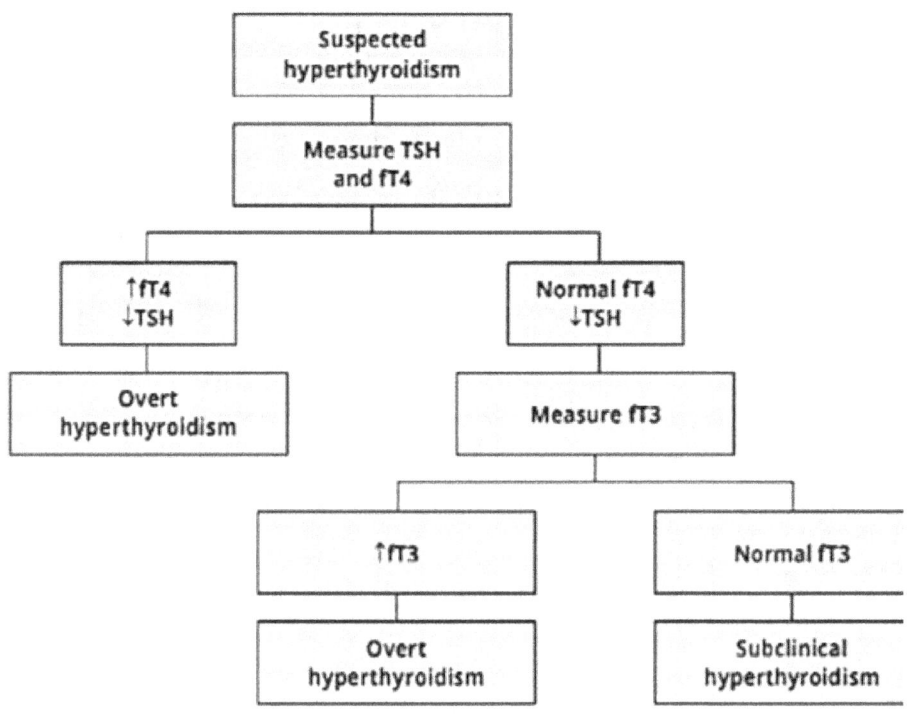

Table 2-1: Grading of Thyroid Vascularity and Pattern via Ultrasound

Grading	Vascular Pattern
Grade 1	No significant intraparenchymal vascularity or minimal spots; low or normal vascularity.
Grade 2	Presence of parenchymal blood flow with uneven, patchy distribution.
Grade 3	Mildly increased color Doppler signal with patchy distribution; elevated vascularity
Grade 4	Markedly increased color Doppler signal with diffuse, homogeneous distribution.

TSH Receptor Antibodies (TRAbs)

TSH receptor antibodies (TRAbs) serve as critical biomarkers in diagnosing Graves' disease. These antibodies not only aid in diagnosis but also help predict the likelihood of relapse and guide long-term treatment strategies for Graves' disease. Two primary methods are available for measuring TRAbs: the competitive binding assay, known as TSH-binding inhibiting immunoglobulin (TBII), and the cell-based bioassay, known as thyroid-stimulating immunoglobulin (TSI). Modern immunoassays predominantly utilize the competitive binding assay (TBII), which detects the presence and concentration of TRAbs but does not assess their functional activity. The third-generation TBII demonstrates a sensitivity and specificity of 99% in diagnosing Graves' disease among hyperthyroid patients. In contrast, highly sensitive cell-based bioassays (TSI) uniquely distinguish between TSH receptor-stimulating antibodies (TSAb) and TSH receptor-blocking antibodies (TBAb).

Figure 2-2: Classification of TRAbs.

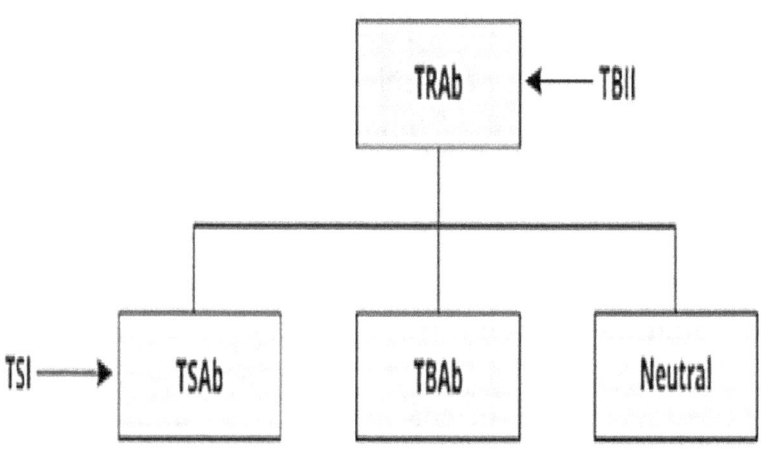

Abbreviations:

- TBII: TSH-binding inhibitory immunoglobulin
- TSI: Thyroid-stimulating immunoglobulin
- TSAb: TSH receptor-stimulating antibody
- TRAb: TSH receptor antibody
- TBAb: TSH receptor-blocking antibody

Thyroid Scintigraphy

Thyroid scintigraphy is the only method capable of evaluating the regional function of the thyroid and identifying autonomously functioning thyroid nodules. This imaging technique is recommended when hyperthyroidism is accompanied by thyroid nodules. However, it is less effective at detecting nodules smaller than 1–1.5 cm in diameter. The American Association of Clinical Endocrinologists (AACE) and the European Thyroid Association (ETA) guidelines identify the radionuclides ^{123}I and ^{99m}Tc as the most commonly used in thyroid scintigraphy. ^{99m}Tc is often favored due to its high availability, lower energy gamma photons, and shorter half-life of six hours, which make it more advantageous compared to ^{123}I.

Recommendations:
- For patients with suspected hyperthyroidism, initial evaluation should include serum TSH and free T4 (fT4) levels. Free T3 (fT3) testing is

recommended if TSH is suppressed but fT4 remains within the normal range.

Figure 2-3: Diagnostic Algorithm for Determining the Cause of Hyperthyroidism.

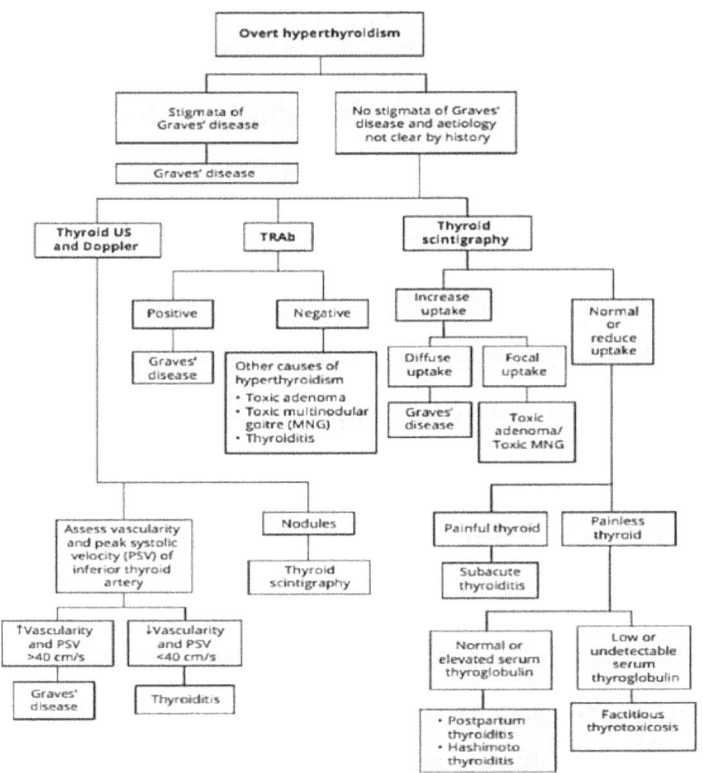

Thyroid Ultrasonography with Color Flow Doppler

Thyroid ultrasonography combined with color flow Doppler provides a reliable method for differentiating between Graves' disease and thyroiditis. It is particularly recommended when scintigraphy is unavailable or not feasible, such as during pregnancy or lactation.

Additional Diagnostic Guidance:
- In cases of overt hyperthyroidism without the typical signs of Graves' disease, testing for TSH receptor antibodies (TRAb) can help differentiate between Graves' disease and other causes of hyperthyroidism.
- Thyroid scintigraphy is advised when a clinical presentation suggests a toxic adenoma, toxic multinodular goiter, or when the diagnosis is uncertain.

How to Treat Hyperthyroidism

For patients with confirmed or highly suspected thyrotoxicosis, treatment with beta-blockers like propranolol, atenolol, or metoprolol can reduce symptoms such as increased heart rate, high systolic blood pressure, muscle weakness, tremors, irritability, emotional instability, and exercise intolerance. Alternatively, calcium channel blockers like verapamil or diltiazem may be used for heart rate control in patients who cannot tolerate or are not candidates for beta-blockers.

Recommendation:
- Beta-adrenergic blockers are recommended for all patients with symptomatic thyrotoxicosis, particularly those who are elderly or have a resting heart rate over 90 beats per minute, or who have coexisting cardiovascular conditions.

How to Treat Graves' Disease (GD)

Once hyperthyroidism is confirmed and identified as due to Graves' disease (GD), patients can choose from three effective and relatively safe initial treatment options: radioactive iodine therapy (^{131}I), antithyroid drugs (ATD), or thyroidectomy. Studies indicate that long-term quality of life (QoL) outcomes are similar across all three treatments.

Radioactive Iodine (RAI) Therapy

RAI is a well-established treatment for hyperthyroidism, generally well-tolerated, and with rare complications, except in cases involving orbitopathy. While thyroid storm is an uncommon occurrence post-RAI administration, RAI may lead to a temporary increase in thyroid hormone levels. To prevent clinical exacerbation of hyperthyroidism, the use of methimazole (MMI) or carbimazole before and after RAI therapy can be considered for patients with severe hyperthyroidism, older patients, or those with significant comorbidities that increase the risk of complications from worsening symptoms.

Table 2:2 Preferred Treatment Modalities for Graves' Hyperthyroidism (Level II)

Treatment Modality	Favorable Clinical Situations	Contraindications
Radioactive Iodine (RAI)	- Women not planning a pregnancy in the near future (within six months, assuming thyroid hormone levels are normal) - Patients with comorbidities that increase the risk of surgery - Individuals with a history of neck surgery or external neck irradiation - Lack of access to a highly experienced thyroid surgeon - Patients who cannot tolerate antithyroid drugs (ATDs) or fail to achieve euthyroidism with ATDs - Patients with periodic	- Pregnancy - Lactation - Coexisting or suspected thyroid cancer - Inability to adhere to radiation safety precautions - Use with caution in women planning pregnancy within 4–6 months

	thyrotoxic hypokalemic paralysis, right heart failure, pulmonary hypertension, or congestive heart failure	
Antithyroid Drugs (ATDs)	- Patients with a high likelihood of remission (especially women with mild disease, small goiters, and negative or low-titer thyroid receptor antibodies) - Pregnant patients - Elderly patients or others with comorbidities that increase surgical risk or limit life expectancy - Individuals in nursing homes or care facilities who may not be able to follow radiation safety guidelines - Patients with a history of neck surgery or irradiation - Lack of access to a	- History of major adverse reactions to ATDs

| | highly experienced thyroid surgeon - Patients with moderate-to-severe active Graves' ophthalmopathy (GO) - Patients needing more rapid biochemical control of their disease | |

Table 2:3 Clinical Contexts Favoring Specific Treatment Modalities for Graves' Hyperthyroidism (Level II)

Treatment Option	Appropriate Clinical Scenarios	Contraindications/ Precautions
Surgery	- Women planning pregnancy within six months, provided	- Lack of access to a highly experienced thyroid surgeon - Pregnancy (relative contraindication): Surgery should be

	thyroid hormone levels are stable - Patients with symptomatic compression or large goiters (>80 g) - Cases with relatively low radioactive iodine uptake - Documented or suspected thyroid malignancy (e.g., suspicious or indeterminate cytology) - Large thyroid nodules (>4 cm) or nonfunctioning/ hypofunctioning nodules on 99mTc pertechnetate	reserved for cases where rapid control of hyperthyroidism is needed, and antithyroid medications cannot be used. Thyroidectomy is ideally avoided during the first and third trimesters due to risks, including teratogenic effects, fetal loss in the first trimester, and preterm labor in the third trimester. The second trimester is considered the safest period for surgery, though it still carries a 4.5%-5.5% risk of preterm labor. - Thyroid surgery during pregnancy also has an increased risk of

	scan - Coexisting hyperparathyroidism requiring surgical intervention - Elevated thyroid-stimulating hormone receptor antibody (TRAb) levels - Patients with moderate-to-severe active Graves' ophthalmopathy (GO)	complications, including hypoparathyroidism and recurrent laryngeal nerve (RLN) injury.

In cases of thyrotoxicosis, particularly in patients with cardiovascular complications such as atrial fibrillation, heart failure, or pulmonary hypertension, as well as those with conditions like renal failure, infection, trauma, poorly managed diabetes mellitus, or cerebrovascular or pulmonary disease, comprehensive medical management is essential. These underlying conditions should be treated to stabilize the patient before proceeding with radioactive iodine (RAI) therapy, whenever feasible.

To minimize potential risks, the use of iodinated radiocontrast should be avoided for at least 4-6 weeks prior to RAI treatment. Additionally, beta-adrenergic blockers should be administered with caution to prepare patients for RAI therapy. Furthermore, methimazole and carbimazole have demonstrated effectiveness in reducing thyroid hormone levels following RAI therapy.

In randomized controlled trials, a special diet is not required before radioactive iodine (RAI) therapy. However, patients should avoid nutritional supplements containing excess iodine, including seaweeds, for at least seven days prior to treatment. For individuals with relatively low radioactive iodine uptake (RAIU), a low-iodine diet may be beneficial to enhance RAI trapping. Patients who might benefit from adjunctive methimazole (MMI) or carbimazole therapy are those who poorly tolerate hyperthyroid symptoms, often presenting with free T4 levels that are 2–3 times the upper limit of normal.

Generally, young and middle-aged patients who are otherwise healthy and compensating well, despite significant biochemical hyperthyroidism, can proceed with RAI therapy without pretreatment. If pretreatment with MMI or carbimazole is required, it should be discontinued before administering RAI. Continuing antithyroid drugs (ATDs) up to 2–3 days before RAIN can help prevent a temporary rise in thyroid hormone levels that typically occurs around six days post-treatment. For elderly patients or those with underlying cardiovascular conditions, resuming MMI or carbimazole 3–7 days after RAI administration should be considered, tapering the dosage as thyroid function stabilizes.

In cases of Graves' disease (GD) where pretreatment with ATDs would have been indicated due to comorbidities or severe symptoms, but where the patient has an allergy to ATDs, the duration of hyperthyroidism may be shortened by administering iodine, such as a saturated solution of potassium iodide (SSKI), starting one week after RAI treatment.

The primary objective of RAI therapy in GD is to control hyperthyroidism by inducing a hypothyroid state. This approach is highly effective as long as an adequate radiation dose is delivered to the thyroid. This goal can be achieved through either a fixed dose method or by calculating the activity based on the size of the thyroid and its RAI uptake capacity. The fixed dose method is straightforward, whereas the calculated dose method requires the determination of two variables: RAI uptake and thyroid size.

Antithyroid Drugs (ATDs)

The aim of ATD therapy is to achieve a euthyroid state as quickly and safely as possible. While ATDs do not cure Graves' hyperthyroidism, they are very effective at controlling it when administered in sufficient doses. Treatment failure is often attributed to nonadherence. Additionally, ATDs may offer immunosuppressive benefits, either by directly reducing thyroid-specific autoimmunity or by alleviating hyperthyroidism, which could help restore immune system regulation.

Carbimazole is rapidly converted to MMI in the bloodstream (10 mg of carbimazole metabolizes to approximately 6 mg of MMI), and both drugs function similarly, proving effective when administered as a single daily dose. Initial MMI doses of 10–30 mg daily are typically used to restore euthyroidism, after which the dosage can be reduced to a maintenance level (usually 5–10 mg daily). The dosage of MMI should be tailored to the severity of thyroid dysfunction, as an insufficient dose may fail to restore euthyroidism in severe cases, while an excessive dose could lead to iatrogenic hypothyroidism in milder cases. Higher doses of MMI are also associated with a greater risk of adverse drug reactions, underscoring the importance of careful dosage management.

To achieve the therapeutic goal of normalizing thyroid function quickly while minimizing adverse effects, careful dosing of methimazole (MMI) is essential. Serum T3 levels should be closely monitored, as some patients may normalize their free T4 levels with MMI but still have elevated serum T3, indicating ongoing thyrotoxicosis. MMI is advantageous due to its once-daily dosing and lower risk of major side effects compared to propylthiouracil (PTU). PTU, having a shorter duration of action, typically requires dosing two or three times per day, starting at 50-150 mg three times daily, depending on the severity of hyperthyroidism. As the patient's clinical status and thyroid function tests normalize, the PTU dose can often be reduced to a maintenance level of 50 mg two or three times daily. In cases requiring faster biochemical control of severe thyrotoxicosis, an initial divided dose of MMI (e.g., 15 or 20 mg twice daily) may be more effective than a single daily dose, as MMI's duration of action can be less than 24 hours.

Adverse Effects of Antithyroid Drugs (ATDs)

Adverse effects of ATDs can be categorized into common, mild allergic reactions and rare, serious allergic or toxic events such as agranulocytosis, vasculitis, or hepatic injury. Minor allergic reactions include pruritus or mild rashes, which are more frequently observed with PTU or higher doses of MMI (30 mg/day) compared to lower doses (15 mg/day). PTU is more commonly associated with hepatotoxicity.

A patient is considered in remission if serum TSH, free T4, and free T3 remain normal for one year after discontinuation of ATD therapy. Remission rates can vary significantly based on geographic location. Meta-analyses suggest that extending ATD therapy beyond 18 months does not improve remission rates in adults. Factors associated with lower remission rates include male gender, smoking (particularly in men), and the presence of large goiters (>80 g). Higher initial MMI doses (60–80 mg/day) do not improve remission rates and are linked to an increased risk of adverse effects, making them not recommended. In cases of relapse after follow-up, treatment options include RAI therapy or surgery.

Surgery

Thyroidectomy offers a high cure rate for hyperthyroidism associated with Graves' disease. Total thyroidectomy has a nearly 0% recurrence rate, whereas subtotal thyroidectomy carries an 8% risk of persistent or recurrent hyperthyroidism within five years. Common complications following near-total or total thyroidectomy include hypocalcemia due to hypoparathyroidism (which can be either transient or permanent), recurrent or superior laryngeal nerve injury (temporary or permanent), postoperative bleeding, and anesthesia-related complications.

Recommendations

- Patients with overt Graves' hyperthyroidism should be treated using one of the following modalities: ATDs, RAI therapy, or thyroidectomy.

- Optimize Comorbidities: Ensure that all comorbid conditions are optimally managed before initiating RAI therapy.

- Consider ATD Pretreatment: In patients at elevated risk of complications due to exacerbation of hyperthyroidism, pretreatment with antithyroid drugs (ATDs) such as methimazole (MMI) should be considered, with discontinuation 2-3 days prior to RAI therapy.

- Administer Adequate RAI: Administer a sufficient dose of radioactive iodine (RAI) in a single session, typically in the range of 10-15 mCi (370-555 MBq), to achieve a hypothyroid state in patients with Graves' disease (GD).

- ATD Resumption Post-RAI: In patients at high risk for complications from worsening hyperthyroidism, resuming ATDs 3-7 days after RAI therapy should be considered.

- Preferred ATD: MMI or carbimazole (CMZ) is the preferred ATD for all patients choosing medication as the primary treatment for GD.

- Patient Education on ATDs: Educate patients about the potential side effects of ATDs and the importance of reporting symptoms such as rash, jaundice, light-colored stools, dark urine, joint pain, abdominal pain, nausea, fatigue, fever, or sore throat to their physician promptly.

- Duration of ATD Therapy: If ATDs are selected as the primary treatment for GD, therapy should be maintained for approximately 12-18 months and then discontinued if TSH levels normalize.

- Post-MMI Hyperthyroidism: If hyperthyroidism recurs after a patient with GD completes a course of MMI, alternative treatments, such as RAI therapy or surgery, should be considered. Continuing low-dose ATD therapy beyond 12-18 months may be an option for patients who do not achieve remission and prefer ongoing medication.

- Surgical Euthyroidism: If surgery is the chosen treatment for GD, patients should be rendered euthyroid before the procedure using ATD pretreatment, with or without beta-blocker therapy.

- Surgical Approach: When surgery is selected as the primary treatment for GD, near-total or total thyroidectomy is the procedure of choice and should be performed by a high-volume thyroid surgeon.

Management of Overt Hyperthyroidism Due to Toxic Multinodular Goiter (TMNG) or Toxic Adenoma (TA)

Two definitive and relatively safe treatment options exist for managing TMNG and TA: RAI therapy and thyroid surgery. Treatment decisions should be based on clinical factors, demographics, and patient preferences. The primary goal of treatment is to rapidly and effectively eliminate the hyperthyroid state. For patients with TMNG, near-total or total thyroidectomy results in less than a 1% risk of treatment failure or the need for repeat intervention, compared to a 20% risk of needing retreatment after RAI therapy. Surgical intervention generally restores euthyroidism within days, though the risk of hypothyroidism and subsequent need for exogenous thyroid hormone therapy is increased.

Following near-total or total thyroidectomy for toxic multinodular goiter (TMNG), patients typically achieve 100% success in eliminating hyperthyroidism. Conversely, for those who undergo radioactive iodine (RAI) therapy, the response rate is about 50% to 60% at three months and rises to 80% by six months. A large study reported a 3% prevalence of hypothyroidism at one year and 64% after 24 years in patients treated with RAI for TMNG, with younger patients (under 50 years of age) being more likely to develop hypothyroidism.

For patients with toxic adenoma (TA), surgical resection, such as ipsilateral thyroid lobectomy or isthmusectomy, results in less than a 1% failure rate, with euthyroidism typically restored within days. Hypothyroidism occurs in 2% to 3% of patients post-lobectomy. In contrast, RAI therapy for TA presents a 6% to 18% risk of persistent hyperthyroidism and a 3% to 5.5% risk of recurrent hyperthyroidism. Approximately 75% of patients respond to RAI therapy within three months, with a response rate of 89% at one year. The risk of developing hypothyroidism after RAI treatment increases over time, especially in patients with antithyroid antibodies or non suppressed TSH levels at the time of therapy.

Table 2-4: Factors Favoring Treatment Modalities for TMNG or TA

Modality	Favors	Contraindications
RAI	- Older age - Significant comorbidities - Prior surgery or neck scarring - Small goiter - Sufficient RAIU for therapy - Lack of access to a high-volume thyroid	- Pregnancy - Lactation - Coexisting thyroid cancer - Inability to follow radiation safety guidelines - Caution in women planning pregnancy within 4–6 months

	surgeon	
Surgery	- Symptoms/signs of compression - Suspected thyroid cancer - Coexisting hyperparathyroidism needing surgery - Large goiter (>80g) - Substernal/retrosternal extension - Insufficient RAIU for therapy - Need for rapid correction	- Severe comorbidities (e.g., cardiopulmonary disease, end-stage cancer) - Lack of access to a high-volume thyroid surgeon - Pregnancy (relative contraindication); surgery only if rapid control of hyperthyroidism is needed and ATDs are not an option

	of thyrotoxicosis	
ATD	- Advanced age - Comorbidities increasing surgical risk - Reduced life expectancy - Poor candidates for ablative therapy	- History of major adverse reactions to ATDs

Recommendations

- Treatment Options for TMNG or TA: Patients with overt TMNG or TA should be treated with either RAI therapy or thyroidectomy. In some cases, long-term, low-dose treatment with methimazole (MMI) may be appropriate.

- Beta-Adrenergic Blockade: Since RAI treatment for TMNG or TA can temporarily exacerbate hyperthyroidism, beta-adrenergic blockers should be considered for patients at an increased risk of complications from worsening hyperthyroidism, such as the elderly or those with comorbid conditions, even if they are asymptomatic.

- Pretreatment with MMI: For patients at a higher risk of complications from worsening hyperthyroidism, particularly the elderly and those with cardiovascular issues or severe hyperthyroidism, pretreatment with MMI before undergoing RAI therapy should be considered, along with beta-adrenergic blockade.

- Resuming ATDs After RAI: In patients at increased risk for complications due to exacerbation of hyperthyroidism, it may be advisable to resume antithyroid drugs (ATDs) 3–7 days following RAI administration.

- Surgical Management of TMNG or TA: For patients with overt hyperthyroidism opting for surgery, it is essential to stabilize thyroid function to a euthyroid state before the procedure using MMI, with or without beta-adrenergic blockers.

- Post-Surgery Management: MMI should be discontinued at the time of surgery, and beta-adrenergic blockers should be gradually tapered off following the procedure.

- Post-Surgical Follow-Up: Persistent or recurrent hyperthyroidism following surgery should prompt an investigation for other potential causes.

- Retreatment After Surgery: RAI therapy should be considered for retreatment in cases of persistent or recurrent hyperthyroidism after inadequate surgery for TMNG or TA.

- Long-Term MMI Treatment: Long-term treatment with MMI may be an option for elderly or chronically ill patients with limited life expectancy, those who are not suitable candidates for surgery or ablative therapy, and those who prefer this approach.

Monitoring Treatment of Hyperthyroidism

Post-RAI Patients: Most patients experience normalization of thyroid function and an improvement in clinical symptoms within 4–8 weeks after RAI therapy. Hypothyroidism can develop as early as four weeks, although it usually occurs between two and six months post-therapy. This transition to hypothyroidism can sometimes be rapid, necessitating thyroid hormone replacement therapy. The timing of hormone replacement should be guided by thyroid function tests, clinical symptoms, and physical examination. Rarely, transient hypothyroidism can occur after RAI therapy, with the potential for complete recovery thereafter.

Monitoring Patients Post-RAI Treatment

In some patients, thyroid function may remain unstable after RAI therapy, with either persistent hyperthyroidism or recurrent thyroid dysfunction. In these cases, the thyroid gland may remain palpable. Beta-blockers prescribed prior to RAI treatment should be gradually tapered off once free T4 and free T3 levels return to the normal range. As thyroid hormone levels stabilize, antithyroid drugs (ATDs) can also be tapered, allowing for an accurate assessment of the RAI response.

Most patients will eventually become hypothyroid, as indicated by a free T4 level below the normal range. At this point, levothyroxine should be initiated. TSH levels may not immediately increase with the onset of hypothyroidism, so they should not be relied upon as the sole indicator for starting levothyroxine therapy. Instead, free T4 levels should guide treatment decisions. It is crucial to avoid overt hypothyroidism, particularly in patients with active Graves' ophthalmopathy (GO).

Once euthyroidism is established, regular thyroid function testing is recommended annually or if symptoms of hypo- or hyperthyroidism emerge. Given that TSH levels may remain suppressed for a month or more after hyperthyroidism resolves, these levels should be interpreted cautiously and in conjunction with free T4 and free T3 levels.

The response to RAI therapy should be monitored through gland size, thyroid function tests, and clinical signs. The aim of retreatment is to achieve control of hyperthyroidism by rendering the patient hypothyroid. Patients with persistently suppressed TSH but normal free T3 and free T4 may not need immediate retreatment but should be monitored closely for relapse or the development of hypothyroidism. For the small percentage of patients whose hyperthyroidism is resistant to multiple rounds of RAI, surgical intervention should be considered.

Monitoring Patients Treated with ATDs

For patients on ATD therapy, regular clinical and biochemical evaluations are essential, and patients must understand the importance of ongoing monitoring. Serum free T4 and free T3 levels should be checked approximately 2–6 weeks after starting treatment, depending on the severity of the thyrotoxicosis. Based on these results, the medication dose should be adjusted. It is particularly important to monitor serum T3, as free T4 levels may normalize even if T3 levels remain elevated.

Serum TSH levels may remain suppressed for several months after starting therapy, so they are not a reliable marker for monitoring treatment in the early stages. Once euthyroid status is achieved, the MMI dose can typically be reduced by 30%–50%, with repeat biochemical testing in 4–6 weeks. After stabilizing euthyroid levels with the lowest effective dose, clinical and laboratory evaluations can be extended to every 2–3 months. For patients on long-term MMI therapy (exceeding 18 months), these intervals can be increased to every six months.

Recommendations

- Follow-Up Monitoring: For patients with Graves' disease (GD), toxic multinodular goiter (TMNG), or toxic adenoma (TA) who have undergone radioiodine (RAI) therapy, initial follow-up within 1–2 months should include assessments of free T4 and, if necessary, free T3 and TSH levels. Continue biochemical monitoring every four to six weeks for up to six months, or until the patient achieves stable hypothyroidism with thyroid hormone replacement.

- Re-Treatment: If hyperthyroidism persists after six months post-RAI therapy, consider additional

RAI treatment. For patients with minimal response three months after initial therapy, further RAI may be warranted.

- Laboratory Monitoring: During febrile illness or at the onset of pharyngitis, obtain a differential white blood cell count for all patients on antithyroid medication.

- Liver Function Assessment: Evaluate liver function and hepatocellular integrity in patients on methimazole (MMI) or propylthiouracil (PTU) who present with symptoms such as pruritic rash, jaundice, light-colored stools, dark urine, joint pain, abdominal pain, bloating, anorexia, nausea, or fatigue.

When to Refer Patients

- Referrals for TMNG or TA: Patients with hyperthyroidism due to TMNG or TA should be referred to facilities with expertise in radioiodine therapy or surgical management.

- Referrals for GD: Patients with GD who remain hyperthyroid despite adequate antithyroid drug (ATD) treatment, or those who relapse after an initial course of ATDs, should be referred to specialized centers with radioiodine facilities or surgical expertise.

- Comorbidities: Hyperthyroid patients with existing or developing comorbid conditions should be referred to a tertiary care center for comprehensive management.

Chapter Three
Subclinical Hyperthyroidism

Definition: Subclinical hyperthyroidism is characterized by suppressed serum TSH levels with normal free T4 and free T3 concentrations. This condition is identified solely through laboratory testing.

Prevalence

The prevalence of subclinical hyperthyroidism ranges from 0.7% in the United States to 2.91% in Europe, influenced by diagnostic criteria, age, sex, TSH assay methods, and iodine intake of the population. A local cross-sectional study reported a prevalence of 2.8%. Other studies indicate a prevalence of up to 1.3% in areas with moderate iodine deficiency and 1.9% in urban men. This condition is more common in older females.

Table 3:1 Causes of Low Serum TSH Levels

Category	Causes
True Subclinical Hyperthyroidism	Endogenous Graves' disease, Multinodular goiter, Autonomous nodule
Exogenous Causes	Intentional thyroxine suppression for thyroid cancer, Unintentional thyroxine replacement for hypothyroidism
Medications	Glucocorticoids, Dopamine, Dobutamine, Octreotide, Amiodarone
Transient Conditions	First trimester of pregnancy, Destructive thyroiditis, Post-radioactive iodine therapy for hyperthyroidism, Severe non-thyroidal illness

Others	Ethnicity (Black Americans), Pituitary or hypothalamic insufficiency, Smoking

Etiology of Subclinical Hyperthyroidism

The aetiology of subclinical hyperthyroidism generally mirrors that of overt hyperthyroidism.

Table 3:2 Association Between Subclinical Hyperthyroidism and Various Outcomes

Event	Prospective Studies	Meta-Analysis	TSH Severity Level	Relationship with Association
Mortality	Probable	√	√	√ (CHD)
Cardiovasc				

ular Events				
Atrial Fibrillation	Probable	√	√	√
Chronic Heart Failure	Possible	√	√	√
Non-fatal Cardiovascular Events	Possible	√	√	√
Bone				
Bone Mass Density	Possible	√		

-Post-menopausal		√		
Premenopausal		√		
Femoral Neck Only		√		
-Total Hip and Lumbar Spine		√		
Fractures	Probable	√	√	√
Stroke	Unclear	√	√	

Cognition	Unclear	√	√	
Symptoms	Possible	√		

Significance of Subclinical Hyperthyroidism

Subclinical hyperthyroidism, characterized by low serum TSH levels with normal free T4 and free T3 concentrations, has been linked to several outcomes. Research indicates a progression to overt hyperthyroidism in 20.3% of patients with TSH levels below 0.1 mIU/L compared to 6.8% in those with TSH levels between 0.1–0.39 mIU/L. Treatment needs vary based on the aetiology, with 9% of subclinical Graves' cases requiring intervention by five years, compared to 21% for multinodular goiter and 61% for autonomous nodules. However, the relationship between non-thyroidal illness and the aetiology of subclinical hyperthyroidism has been shown to be inconclusive.

Atrial Fibrillation

Subclinical hyperthyroidism has been linked to atrial fibrillation in several prospective studies. Both prospective studies and meta-analyses indicate a correlation between the severity of TSH levels and the risk of atrial fibrillation.

Chronic Heart Failure

While some prospective studies suggest a connection between subclinical hyperthyroidism and chronic heart failure, the evidence is mixed. A meta-analysis by Gencer et al. reported a hazard ratio (HR) of 1.46 (95% CI, 0.94–2.27; $p>0.05$), indicating a possible association, though statistical significance was not achieved. The data suggest that lower TSH levels (<0.1 mIU/L) might be linked to heart failure.

Non-fatal Cardiovascular Events

Most prospective studies show an increased hazard ratio for non-fatal cardiovascular events in individuals with subclinical hyperthyroidism, though not always reaching statistical significance. An individual participant meta-analysis by Collet found an HR of 1.21 (95% CI, 0.99–1.46) for coronary heart disease events, with no clear association of lower TSH levels (<0.1 mIU/L) with higher risk. Conversely, a meta-analysis by Li-bo Yang reported an HR of 1.19 (95% CI, 1.10–1.28; p<0.05), suggesting a significant association.

Fractures

The Busselton Health Study found no association between subclinical hyperthyroidism and fractures, whereas the Health, Aging, and Body Composition Study indicated a significant association. An individual participant data meta-analysis by Blum revealed increased risk for fractures, including hip fractures (HR 1.36; 95% CI, 1.13–1.64), any fractures (HR 1.28; 95% CI, 1.06–1.53), and spine fractures (HR

1.51; 95% CI, 0.93–2.45). Lower TSH levels were associated with a higher fracture risk.

Bone Mineral Density (BMD)

The Rotterdam Study identified decreased BMD in patients with subclinical hyperthyroidism, whereas the Cardiovascular Health Study did not. A meta-analysis by Segna et al. reported greater BMD loss at the femoral neck in individuals with subclinical hyperthyroidism, particularly in those with TSH <0.10 mIU/L. Ruifei Yang et al. observed BMD reduction primarily at the femoral neck and total hip, predominantly among women.

Stroke

A prospective study by Parle suggested an increased risk of stroke in subclinical hyperthyroidism, but this was not supported by another study by Cappola. A meta-analysis by Chaker found no significant association between subclinical hyperthyroidism and stroke.

Cognition

Kalmijn's study suggested an increased risk of dementia in individuals with subclinical hyperthyroidism. In contrast, Formiga's study found no such association. However, a meta-analysis by Rieben indicated a significant link between subclinical hyperthyroidism and dementia, with a hazard ratio (HR) of 1.67 (95% CI, 1.04–2.69).

Symptoms

Research by Stott revealed that individuals with subclinical hyperthyroidism had higher mean Wayne scores compared to those with normal thyroid function.

Recommendations

- Assessments: Regular evaluations using ECG, echocardiography, and bone mineral density tests are advisable for patients with subclinical hyperthyroidism.

Benefits of Treatment for Subclinical Hyperthyroidism

Currently, there are no large randomized controlled trials assessing the impact of treatment on mortality, cardiovascular events, fractures, stroke, or cognitive function in subclinical hyperthyroidism. However, several smaller studies have explored the effects of treatment on symptoms, cardiac structure and function, heart rate, body composition, and bone mineral density.

Table 3:4 Benefits of Subclinical Hyperthyroidism Treatment

Outcome Measures	Treatment Modality	Benefits
Symptom	Methimaz	Yes

s	ole (83)	
	Propylthiouracil, RAI (84)	Yes
Cardiac Function, Rates, Structure	Methimazole (83)	Yes
	Propylthiouracil, RAI (84)	Yes
	Methimazole (86)	Yes
	Propylthiouracil (88)	Yes
Bone Mass Density	Propylthiouracil, RAI (84)	Yes
	RAI (85)	Yes
	Methimazole (86)	Yes

	RAI, Thyroidectomy (87)	Yes
Body Composition	RAI, Thyroidectomy (87)	Yes

Beta-Blocker Use in Thyroxine Suppressive Therapy

Bisoprolol, a beta-blocker, has been employed in patients undergoing thyroxine suppressive therapy. It has been effective in alleviating symptoms, decreasing heart rate, and reducing left ventricular hypertrophy.

Management of Patients with Low TSH Levels

Figure 3:1 Flowchart for Evaluating the Causes of Low TSH Levels. (Adapted from 4 Level II)

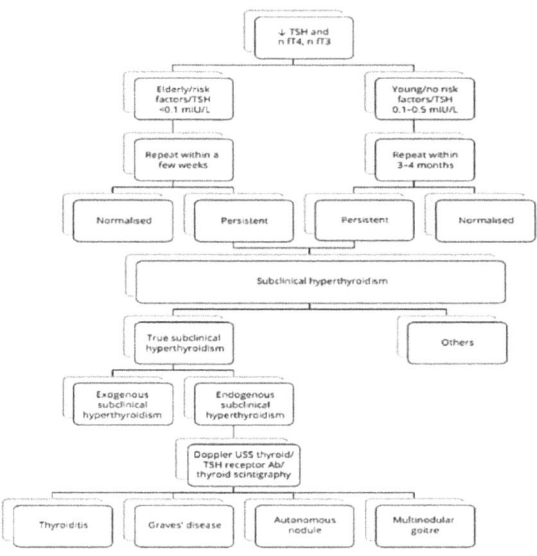

Treatment of Subclinical Hyperthyroidism

Current evidence suggests that subclinical hyperthyroidism may contribute to atrial fibrillation and could potentially increase the risks of mortality and fractures. It might also be linked to heart failure and cardiovascular events. However, its role in stroke and dementia remains uncertain. Existing studies primarily evaluate treatment outcomes through surrogate markers, such as symptoms, cardiac structure and function, bone mineral density, and body composition. The American Thyroid Association's 2016 guidelines provide recommendations for managing subclinical hyperthyroidism.

Table 3:5 Considerations for Treating Subclinical Hyperthyroidism [Adapted from 4 Level II]

Factor	TSH (<0.1 mIU/L)	TSH (0.1–0.4 mIU/L)
Age >65 years	Yes	Consider treatment
Age <65 years with comorbidities	Yes	Consider treatment

Heart disease	Yes	Consider treatment
Osteoporosis	Yes	Consider treatment
Menopausal, not on estrogens or bisphosphonates	Yes	Menopausal, not on estrogens or bisphosphonatesYesConsider treatment
Hyperthyroid symptoms	Yes	Consider treatment
Age <65	Conside	Observ

| years, asymptomatic | r treatment | e |

Recommendations

- Treatment Considerations: Initiate treatment for patients with subclinical hyperthyroidism who are either over 65 years of age, have comorbidities (such as cardiac disease or osteoporosis), or have a TSH level below 0.1 mIU/L.

- Younger Patients: For those under 65 years, without comorbidities, and with a TSH between 0.1 and 0.5 mIU/L who are asymptomatic, observation is recommended rather than immediate treatment.

- Symptomatic Patients: Beta-blockers should be prescribed to manage symptoms in individuals with symptomatic subclinical hyperthyroidism.

- Treatment Strategy: When treatment is warranted, it should follow established guidelines for overt hyperthyroidism, tailored to the specific aetiology.

- Initial Treatment: Anti-thyroid drugs should be the first-line therapy for subclinical hyperthyroidism, regardless of its cause.

Figure 3:2 Treatment Decision-Making Process for Subclinical Hyperthyroidism [Adapted from 4 Level II]

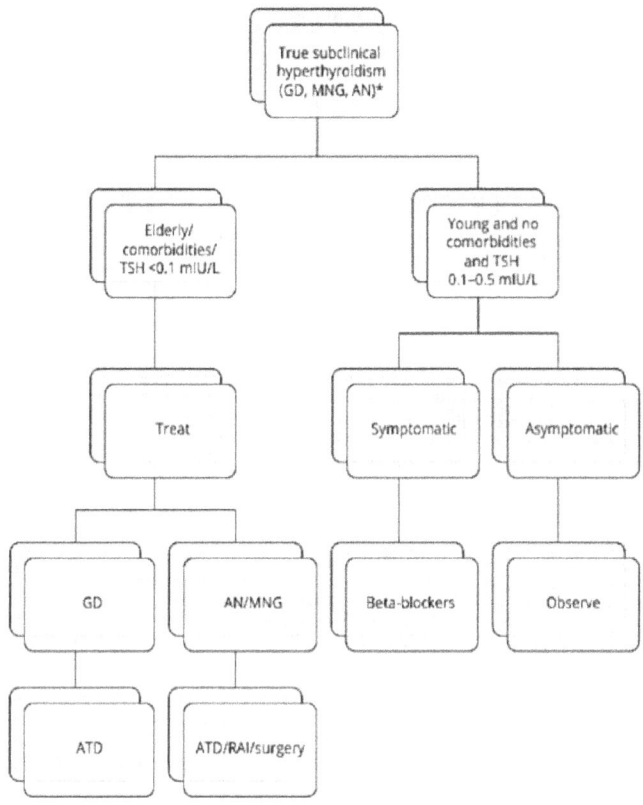

- Radioactive iodine therapy should be considered for patients with persistent and worsening subclinical hyperthyroidism caused by autonomous nodules or multinodular goiter.

- Surgery should be considered only for individuals experiencing compressive symptoms, such as dysphagia or shortness of breath, or if there is suspicion of malignancy.

Hypothyroidism
Overt Hypothyroidism

Clinical and Biochemical Goals for Levothyroxine Replacement in Primary Hypothyroidism

The primary goals for levothyroxine replacement therapy in primary hypothyroidism are to achieve euthyroidism and normalize circulating levels of thyroid-stimulating hormone (TSH) and thyroid hormones.

Recommendations:

- Levothyroxine is the preferred and standard treatment for hypothyroidism.
- The therapy aims to:
    1. Resolve signs and symptoms of hypothyroidism, including biological and physiological markers.

2. Normalize serum TSH and improve thyroid hormone levels.

3. Prevent iatrogenic thyrotoxicosis or overtreatment, especially in elderly patients.

Assessing Adequacy of Levothyroxine Replacement

Clinical signs and symptoms such as cold intolerance and dry skin are neither sensitive nor specific for assessing the adequacy of levothyroxine replacement, as they can overlap with other conditions. Therefore, these symptoms should not be used in isolation to judge treatment adequacy. Instead, longitudinal assessment of clinical symptoms should be combined with serum TSH and thyroid hormone levels, taking into account comorbidities and other possible causes.

Recommendations

Levothyroxine Administration Timing

- Levothyroxine should be taken on an empty stomach—either 1 hour before breakfast or at bedtime, ensuring it is taken at least 3 hours after the last meal of the day. This is because food can impair absorption. However, to improve compliance, it may be beneficial to instruct patients to take it consistently before breakfast.

Recommendation

- To prevent interference with levothyroxine absorption, it is recommended to separate its administration from other potentially conflicting medications and supplements. A separation of four hours is advised.

Medications and Supplements Affecting Levothyroxine Absorption

Various studies indicate that the absorption of levothyroxine can be impaired by certain medications and beverages, such as coffee.

- Bile acid sequestrants (e.g., cholestyramine, colestipol, colesevelam)
- Sucralfate
- Cation exchange resins (e.g., Kayexalate)
- Oral bisphosphonates
- Proton pump inhibitors
- Raloxifene
- Multivitamins containing ferrous sulfate or calcium carbonate
- Ferrous sulfate
- Phosphate binders (e.g., sevelamer, aluminum hydroxide)
- Calcium salts (e.g., carbonate, citrate, acetate)
- Chromium picolinate
- Charcoal
- Orlistat
- Ciprofloxacin
- H2 receptor antagonists

Conditions and Diet

- Malabsorption syndromes (e.g., celiac disease, jejunoileal bypass surgery, biliary cirrhosis, achlorhydria)

- Diet-related factors (e.g., ingestion with a meal, grapefruit juice, espresso coffee, high-fiber diet, soybean formula for infants, soy)

Gastrointestinal Conditions Affecting Levothyroxine Dosage

Certain gastrointestinal disorders can impact levothyroxine absorption or serum TSH levels, often through alterations in gastric acidity. Research has demonstrated that the need for levothyroxine may decrease following treatment for H. pylori infection and implementation of a gluten-free diet in individuals with celiac disease. Conversely, levothyroxine absorption seems unaffected by Roux-en-Y gastric bypass and other similar procedures, as the ileum remains the primary site of absorption. Additionally, autoimmune atrophic gastritis is commonly observed in older patients with hypothyroidism and Hashimoto's thyroiditis.

Recommendation:

- Assess gastrointestinal disorders (e.g., H. pylori infection, atrophic gastritis, and celiac disease) in patients requiring significantly higher doses of levothyroxine. If these conditions are identified and treated, reassess thyroid function and adjust the levothyroxine dosage as necessary.

Medications Affecting Levothyroxine Requirements

Medications that impact levothyroxine metabolism or alter thyroxine-binding globulin levels may necessitate adjustments in levothyroxine dosage. Significant increases in levothyroxine requirements have been observed in patients taking tyrosine kinase inhibitors, such as imatinib and sunitinib.

Recommendation:
- Reevaluate serum TSH levels when initiating or discontinuing estrogen, androgens, or medications that affect thyroxine metabolism, including tyrosine kinase inhibitors. Monitoring

is also recommended when starting drugs that enhance hepatic metabolism of T4 and T3, such as antiepileptics (e.g., phenobarbital, phenytoin, carbamazepine), rifampicin, or sertraline.

Factors Influencing Levothyroxine Dose

Several factors can influence the levothyroxine dose required to achieve target serum TSH levels. The initial levothyroxine dose should be determined based on the following considerations:

[Detailed factors will follow, potentially including patient age, body weight, underlying health conditions, and specific thyroid function test results.]

Factors Influencing Levothyroxine Dosage

Several factors determine the appropriate levothyroxine dosage needed to normalize serum TSH levels. Key considerations include:

- Body Weight: The standard starting dose is 1.6 µg/kg of body weight for significant TSH elevations. For milder hypothyroidism, a lower starting dose of 25–50 µg/day is often sufficient.
- Lean Body Mass: Adjustments may be needed based on lean body mass.
- Pregnancy Status: Pregnant patients may require dosage adjustments.
- Aetiology of Hypothyroidism: The underlying cause of hypothyroidism can impact dosing requirements.
- Degree of TSH Elevation: Higher TSH levels generally necessitate higher doses.
- Age: Dosage may vary with age, particularly in elderly patients.
- General Medical Condition: Conditions like cardiac disease can influence dosage needs.
- Serum TSH Goal: The target TSH level should be tailored to the patient's clinical situation.

Initiating and Adjusting Levothyroxine Therapy

When starting levothyroxine therapy, dosage should be based on serum TSH levels and body weight. For markedly elevated TSH, a full replacement dose of 1.6 µg/kg is recommended, whereas milder cases may require 25–50 µg/day. Concurrent medications may also affect the required dose.

Recommendation:
- Begin levothyroxine therapy with either a full or partial replacement dose, adjusting gradually based on serum TSH levels. Reassess and adjust doses in response to significant weight changes, pregnancy, and aging. Serum TSH levels should be evaluated 4–8 weeks following any dosage adjustment.

Risks of Excessive Levothyroxine

Overdosing on levothyroxine can lead to iatrogenic thyrotoxicosis, which may cause atrial fibrillation and increased bone loss, potentially leading to osteoporosis. It is crucial to avoid excessive thyroid hormone levels and very low serum TSH, especially in older individuals and postmenopausal women.

Reference: See the sections on subclinical hyperthyroidism and hyperthyroidism in the elderly for further details.

Risks of Inadequate Levothyroxine

Insufficient levothyroxine can negatively impact serum lipid profiles and exacerbate cardiovascular disease. Ensuring adequate levothyroxine doses to achieve normal serum TSH levels is essential to mitigate these risks.

Reference: Consult the section on the effects of subclinical hypothyroidism for additional information.

Managing Levothyroxine Allergy or Intolerance

Allergic reactions to levothyroxine are rare but have been reported, particularly related to tablet dyes.

Recommendation:

- For patients experiencing intolerance or allergic reactions to levothyroxine, alternative formulations or adjustments should be considered.

Recommendation:
- If a patient appears to be allergic or intolerant to levothyroxine, consider adjusting the dosage or switching to alternative formulations, such as gel capsules. Additionally, addressing any coexisting conditions like iron-deficiency anemia may help. In some cases, a referral to an allergist might be useful to identify other potential allergens that could be causing the reaction mistakenly attributed to levothyroxine.

Management of Levothyroxine Therapy in Cases of Elevated TSH Due to Nonadherence:

Recommendation:
- For patients with elevated serum TSH levels who are presumed nonadherent but who can absorb levothyroxine properly, administering the full weekly dose in a single weekly dose might

be effective. This method has been demonstrated to safely and effectively reduce TSH levels in such cases.

Biochemical Goals for Levothyroxine Replacement in Secondary Hypothyroidism:

Recommendation:
- The main biochemical target for patients with secondary hypothyroidism is to maintain serum free thyroxine (fT4) levels in the upper half of the reference range. However, for older patients or those with additional health conditions, the target level may need to be adjusted to minimize the risk of complications associated with excess thyroid hormone.

Approach for Patients with Normal Serum TSH but Persistent Symptoms:

Recommendation:
- For patients who have normal serum TSH levels but continue to experience symptoms, particularly those with Hashimoto's thyroiditis,

it is important to recognize that hypothyroidism might be just one contributing factor. Additional factors, such as psychological distress or other underlying conditions, should be evaluated and addressed as they may also contribute to the persistent symptoms.

Addressing Unmet Needs in Levothyroxine-Treated Hypothyroid Patients:

Recommendation:
- Acknowledge and address the persistent symptoms reported by patients receiving levothyroxine, despite having normal serum TSH levels. Evaluate these symptoms for potential alternative causes to provide comprehensive care.

Biological Basis for Persistent Complaints in Levothyroxine-Treated Hypothyroid Patients:

Recommendation:
- Persistent symptoms in patients with hypothyroidism treated with levothyroxine, even

with normal TSH levels, may be linked to the underlying autoimmune nature of their thyroid condition. Autoimmune thyroid diseases, such as Hashimoto's thyroiditis and post-thyroid ablation, are frequently associated with other autoimmune disorders, including rheumatoid arthritis and various other conditions. These associated autoimmune diseases might contribute to ongoing symptoms. Therefore, screening for additional autoimmune disorders is recommended for patients with autoimmune thyroid conditions who present with new or unresolved symptoms.

When to Involve Endocrinologists in Hypothyroidism Care:

Recommendation:
- Consultation with an endocrinologist is advisable for:
  - Pediatric patients, including children and infants
  - Individuals with challenges in achieving and maintaining euthyroidism

- Pregnant women and those planning pregnancy
- Patients with underlying cardiac conditions
- Those with thyroid gland abnormalities such as goiter or nodules
- Individuals with concurrent endocrine disorders, including adrenal or pituitary issues
- Cases with atypical thyroid function test results
- Situations involving unusual causes of hypothyroidism, such as drug-induced conditions or therapy with tyrosine kinase inhibitors

Management of Levothyroxine Therapy in Hospitalized Patients:

Recommendation:
- When managing hospitalized patients with pre-existing hypothyroidism, adjustments to levothyroxine therapy should be based on clinical and biochemical evaluations of hypothyroidism, the presence of active comorbidities, and specific aspects of

levothyroxine administration, such as dosage, timing, and factors affecting absorption.

Recommended Levothyroxine Formulation and Administration Route

Recommendation:
- Oral levothyroxine is the preferred method of administration. If oral administration is not feasible, alternative enteral routes may be used. In cases where enteral administration is contraindicated or there is significant concern about malabsorption, intravenous levothyroxine should be considered, typically at approximately 75% of the oral dose.

- Intravenous levothyroxine may be utilized if enteral absorption is inadequate or if enteral administration is contraindicated. This should be done at about 75% of the oral dose, assuming the oral dosage previously achieved euthyroidism. This approach should continue until internal absorption improves.

Evaluation for Adrenal Insufficiency in Hospitalized Patients:

Recommendation:
- Consider screening for adrenal insufficiency in hospitalized patients starting levothyroxine therapy. If clinical or biochemical signs suggest adrenal insufficiency, empiric treatment should be initiated.

Subclinical Hypothyroidism

Causes of Subclinical Hypothyroidism:

The predominant cause of subclinical hypothyroidism is chronic autoimmune thyroiditis, also known as Hashimoto's disease. Other less common causes include:
- Post-treatment conditions such as radioactive iodine therapy, subtotal thyroidectomy, and the use of antithyroid drugs.

- External factors like head and neck surgeries, radiation therapy, iodine deficiency, and untreated primary adrenal insufficiency.
- Medication-related issues with drugs like lithium, iodine, and amiodarone.
- Secondary causes such as hypopituitarism and idiopathic or congenital factors.
- Transient elevations of TSH can occur with subacute or painless thyroiditis, following L-thyroxine withdrawal, or during recovery from significant nonthyroidal illnesses. It is advisable to repeat TSH measurements every two to three months to confirm a persistent elevation.

Diagnosis and Management of Subclinical Hypothyroidism

Subclinical hypothyroidism is diagnosed through laboratory tests. It is characterized by an elevated serum TSH concentration while serum free T4 (fT4) and T3 levels remain within their reference ranges. To confirm the diagnosis, repeat TSH testing is recommended within two to three months due to the potential for transient

TSH abnormalities caused by factors such as subacute thyroiditis, L-thyroxine withdrawal, recovery from severe nonthyroidal illnesses, or use of certain medications like lithium and amiodarone. Patients with subclinical hypothyroidism may exhibit few or no clear clinical signs of thyroid dysfunction. TSH levels generally show a log-linear relationship with circulating thyroid hormones. The standard reference range for serum TSH is 0.40–4.2 mIU/L. Testing for anti-TPO antibodies can help assess the risk of progression to overt hypothyroidism.

Spontaneous recovery from subclinical hypothyroidism has been observed, particularly in individuals with negative antithyroid antibodies and serum TSH levels below 10 mIU/L, especially within the first two years following diagnosis.

Recommendations:

- Subclinical hypothyroidism is characterized by an elevated serum TSH level with normal serum free T4 (fT4) levels.
- Elevated TSH levels should be confirmed with repeat measurements to establish a definitive diagnosis.
- Measuring anti-TPO antibodies can help assess the risk of progression to overt hypothyroidism.

Complications and Progression of Subclinical Hypothyroidism:

Although subclinical hypothyroidism often presents with minimal symptoms, research indicates some patients do experience mild thyroid failure. The Colorado Thyroid Disease Prevalence study, involving 25,862 participants, found subtle differences in symptoms such as drier skin, poorer memory, slower thinking, and increased tiredness among those with subclinical hypothyroidism compared to euthyroid controls.

The Tromsø study, with 154 controls and 89 patients with subclinical hypothyroidism (TSH between 3.5 and 10.0 mIU/L), found that only tiredness was significantly different between groups, suggesting that while some patients do show symptoms, they may be mild.

Subclinical hypothyroidism often progresses to overt hypothyroidism. A study by Gerold Huber, Jean-Jacques Staub, and colleagues tracked 82 women with subclinical hypothyroidism over a mean period of 9.2 years. The 10-year incidence of overt hypothyroidism was 0% for those with initial TSH levels of 4 to 6 μIU/mL, 42.8% for those with levels of 6 to 12 μIU/mL, and 76.9% for those with levels exceeding 12 μIU/mL. The risk of progression was notably higher with elevated baseline TSH levels. Additionally, the presence of anti-TPO antibodies correlated with an increased risk of progressing to overt hypothyroidism. However, some patients may experience normalization of their thyroid function without progression.

Progression and Lipid Associations in Subclinical Hypothyroidism:

A TSH level exceeding 10 mIU/L is associated with a higher risk of progressing to overt hypothyroidism, while a level below 6 mIU/L indicates a lower risk of progression. In a study involving individuals aged over 55, with an average follow-up of 32 months, 52% of those with initial TSH levels below 10 mIU/L experienced normalization of their TSH levels.

Subclinical hypothyroidism is linked to elevated total cholesterol (TC), low-density lipoprotein cholesterol (LDL-C), and triglycerides (TG), all of which generally decrease with appropriate treatment. Increased levels of TC, LDL-C, and TG are associated with a heightened risk of coronary heart disease (CHD); hence, careful monitoring of cardiovascular health in patients with subclinical hypothyroidism is essential. A meta-analysis of 40,516 participants provided weak evidence connecting high-density lipoprotein cholesterol (HDL-C) levels with subclinical hypothyroidism.

Systematic reviews and meta-analyses indicate that the risk of CHD events rises with higher TSH levels, particularly when TSH levels are ≥10.0 mIU/L. Minimal TSH variations between 4.5 and 6.9 mIU/L do not appear to correlate with CHD events. Additionally, no significant link has been found between subclinical hypothyroidism and fracture risk, nor with symptoms of anxiety, depression, or cognitive dysfunction.

Chapter Four
Thyroid Nodules/Goitre

A thyroid nodule is defined as a discrete lesion within the thyroid gland, resulting from abnormal focal growth of thyroid cells. Typically, thyroid nodules are benign, including hyperplastic or colloid nodules and follicular adenomas. Malignancy occurs in only 5%–10% of nodules. A non-toxic goitre is characterized by thyroid enlargement due to uniform or selective growth of thyroid tissue without the presence of hyperthyroidism or hypothyroidism, and not caused by inflammation or neoplasia.

Prevalence of Thyroid Nodules and Goitre

The prevalence of goiter, whether diffuse or nodular, varies greatly depending on the population's iodine intake. Goitre may be endemic, primarily due to iodine deficiency, or it can occur sporadically. Using ultrasonography, studies have found that up to 30%–50% of an unselected adult population may have goiter, with higher prevalence in regions with iodine deficiency and among older individuals.

Thyroid nodules are a frequent clinical finding. In large population-based studies, the prevalence of thyroid nodules detected by physical examination is estimated to be between 4% and 7%. Imaging techniques, especially ultrasonography, reveal up to ten times more nodules than physical examination alone, most of which are benign. Ultrasonography studies report detection rates for non-palpable thyroid nodules ranging from 20% to 75% in the general population. The prevalence of thyroid nodules is higher in older adults, females, and individuals from iodine-deficient areas.

Typical Clinical Presentation of Thyroid Nodules and Goitre

Thyroid nodules generally do not lead to abnormal thyroid hormone levels and are often asymptomatic. Patients typically present with a neck lump or swelling, with approximately 70% of those with sporadic nontoxic goiter reporting neck discomfort. Concerns about cosmetic appearance and potential malignancy are also common.

Large goiters can compress or displace the trachea, esophagus, and neck vessels, potentially causing compressive symptoms such as inspiratory stridor, dysphagia, or a choking sensation. Compression of the recurrent laryngeal nerve may result in hoarseness of voice due to vocal cord paralysis, which is often associated with thyroid malignancy.

Clinical Evaluation of Thyroid Nodules and Goitre

The primary goal of evaluating a thyroid nodule is to distinguish between malignant and benign conditions. Most nodules are benign and asymptomatic. The initial evaluation should include a thorough history and physical examination.

Historical factors suggestive of benign conditions include:
- Family history of Hashimoto's thyroiditis or benign thyroid conditions
- Symptoms consistent with hypothyroidism or hyperthyroidism
- Sudden nodule enlargement with pain or tenderness, indicating possible cyst or localized thyroiditis

Historical features indicative of potential malignancy include:
- Age extremes (under 20 years or over 60 years)
- Male gender
- History of external neck radiation during childhood or adolescence
- Rapid growth of the nodule
- Recent changes in speaking, breathing, or swallowing
- Family history of thyroid cancer or Multiple Endocrine Neoplasia type 2

Physical signs that may suggest malignancy include:
- Firm or hard nodule consistency
- Irregular shape
- Fixation to surrounding tissues
- Vocal cord paralysis
- Suspicious regional lymphadenopathy

The presence of multiple thyroid nodules does not necessarily reduce the risk of thyroid cancer. In patients with multiple nodules, the reduction in the likelihood of malignancy is roughly proportional to the number of nodules present. While thyroid cancer is frequently found in the dominant nodule, it can also occur in one-third of cases in a non-dominant nodule.

Recommendations:
- A comprehensive medical history should include:
  - Personal or family history of thyroid disease or cancer
    - Previous exposure to head, neck, or whole-body irradiation

- History of surgery, especially in the head, neck, or upper esophagus/thorax regions
- Rate of growth of the neck mass
- Use of iodine-containing medications or supplements
- Symptoms indicative of thyroid dysfunction (hypothyroidism or hyperthyroidism)
- Symptoms such as dysphagia, dysphonia, or dyspnea, which may indicate compression or invasion of nearby structures
- The physical examination should involve a detailed assessment of:
- Thyroid gland size and texture
- Location, consistency, size, and number of thyroid nodules
- Presence of tenderness or pain in the neck
- Enlargement of central and lateral cervical lymph nodes

Ultrasound Evaluation of Thyroid Nodules and Goitre

For the assessment of a nodular goiter, ultrasound (US) is the preferred imaging method. It provides crucial information on the characteristics of nodules, including their potential malignancy risk and size, which helps determine the need for Fine Needle Aspiration Biopsy (FNAB).

Recommendation:
- Patients with a suspected thyroid nodule or nodular goiter, or those with incidental findings of a thyroid nodule on other imaging studies, should undergo a dedicated thyroid and neck ultrasound. This should include evaluation of the thyroid and both central and lateral neck compartments.

Ultrasound is considered the gold standard for evaluating the size of thyroid nodules and the characteristics of the thyroid parenchyma, including whether it is homogeneous or heterogeneous.

To accurately assess thyroid nodules and cervical lymph nodes in both central and lateral compartments, specific characteristics must be evaluated. These include the nodule's composition (proportion of solid to cystic areas), echogenicity, shape (notably if taller than wide), margins, and the presence of any echogenic foci.

Ultrasound Description of Thyroid Nodules

A consistent and structured approach to evaluating and documenting thyroid nodules via ultrasound is essential to ensure accurate diagnosis, risk stratification, and subsequent management. The American College of Radiology (ACR) introduced the TI-RADS (Thyroid Imaging Reporting and Data System) in 2017, a widely accepted, user-friendly system. This structured reporting method improves the assessment of malignancy risk in thyroid nodules, aiding in the decision-making process regarding whether fine needle aspiration (FNA) or surgery is necessary. The use of this system also minimizes unnecessary invasive procedures and enhances communication between radiologists, physicians, and patients.

For patients presenting with four or more nodules, only the four nodules with the highest TI-RADS scores should be evaluated, reported, and monitored. Follow-up should be based on the nodule with the highest TI-RADS score. Other nodules should be re-evaluated via ultrasound. An increase in nodule size is considered significant if there is a 20% and 2 mm increase in two dimensions or a 50% increase in volume. If the TI-RADS score increases on subsequent scans, another follow-up scan should be scheduled the following year. If no changes in size or TI-RADS classification are observed over a five-year period, ultrasound monitoring can be discontinued, as this stability indicates a benign nature.

Fine Needle Aspiration Biopsy (FNAB) of Thyroid Nodules

Fine needle aspiration biopsy (FNAB) remains the primary method for diagnosing thyroid cancer, with high sensitivity and specificity. This procedure is generally safe and straightforward, requiring an adequate sample that includes at least five or six groups of 10-15 well-preserved cells. Ultrasound guidance is recommended during FNAB, especially for nodules with a higher risk of non-diagnostic results (e.g., those with more than 25-50% cystic content) or sampling errors (e.g., non-palpable or posteriorly located nodules). FNAB is advised for nodules classified as TR3-TR5 under the ACR TI-RADS 2017 management algorithm:

- TR1: No FNA needed
- TR2: No FNA needed

ACR-TI RADS 2017 Structured Reporting System for Thyroid Nodule Ultrasound

Composition (Select One)
- Cystic or Almost Completely Cystic: 0 points
- Spongiform: 0 points
- Mixed Cystic and Solid: 1 point
- Solid or Almost Completely Solid: 2 points

Echogenicity (Select One)

- Anechoic: 0 points
- Hyperechoic or Isoechoic: 1 point
- Hypoechoic: 2 points
- Very Hypoechoic: 3 points

Shape (Select One)
- Wider-Than-Tall: 0 points
- Taller-Than-Wide: 3 points

Margin (Select One)
- Smooth: 0 points
- Ill-Defined: 0 points
- Lobulated or Irregular: 2 points
- Extrathyroidal Extension: 3 points

Echogenic Foci (Select All That Apply)
- Macrocalcifications: 1 point
- Peripheral (Rim) Calcifications: 2 points
- Punctate Echogenic Foci: 3 points
- None or Large Comet-Tail Artifacts: 0 points

TI-RADS Classification Based on Total Points
- 0 Points: TR1 - Benign, No FNA
- 2 Points: TR2 - Not Suspicious, No FNA

- 3 Points: TR3 - Mildly Suspicious, FNA if ≥2.5 cm, Follow if ≥1.5 cm
- 4 to 6 Points: TR4 - Moderately Suspicious, FNA if ≥1.5 cm, Follow if ≥1 cm
- 7 Points or More: TR5 - Highly Suspicious, FNA if ≥1 cm, Follow if ≥0.5 cm

Additional Guidelines

1. Spongiform Nodules: Composed predominantly (>50%) of small cystic spaces. No further points are assigned in other categories.
2. Mixed Cystic and Solid Nodules: Points should be assigned based on the predominant solid component.
3. Anechoic Nodules: Applies to nodules that are entirely or almost entirely cystic.
4. Echogenicity Considerations: Hyperechoic, isoechoic, and hypoechoic classifications should be made in comparison to adjacent thyroid tissue. Very hypoechoic nodules are darker than the surrounding strap muscles.

5. Shape Consideration: The taller-than-wide classification is based on the transverse view of the nodule, with the height measured parallel to the sound beam and the width perpendicular.

6. Margin Definitions: Lobulated margins refer to protrusions into adjacent tissues, while irregular margins are jagged or spiculated. Extrathyroidal extension signifies invasive malignancy.

7. Echogenic Foci: Large comet-tail artifacts (>1 mm) typically appear in cystic nodules. Microcalcifications create acoustic shadowing, while peripheral calcifications form complete or incomplete rings along the nodule's margin. Punctate echogenic foci may exhibit small comet-tail artifacts.

Follow-Up and Fine Needle Aspiration (FNA) Guidelines for TR3, TR4, and TR5 Nodules:

- TR3:
  - Follow-Up: Recommended for nodules ≥1.5 cm at 1, 3, and 5 years.
  - FNAB: Indicated for nodules ≥2.5 cm.

- TR4:
  - Follow-Up: Suggested for nodules ≥1.0 cm at 1, 2, 3, and 5 years.
  - FNAB: Required for nodules ≥1.5 cm.

- TR5:
  - Follow-Up: Initiated for nodules ≥0.5 cm, with annual monitoring for up to 5 years.
  - FNAB: Necessary for nodules ≥1.0 cm.

#Approach for Multiple Nodules:

When multiple nodules are present, biopsy should be performed on the two nodules with the highest ACR TI-RADS classifications. Additionally, suspicious cervical lymph nodes (in levels II, III, IV, and VI) should be evaluated. If metastatic lymph nodes are suspected, FNA may be warranted for subcentimeter nodules with a TI-RADS grade of 4 or 5, or the nodule with the highest TI-RADS score, irrespective of its size.

Cytology Reports for FNAB Samples of Thyroid Nodules

A standardized system is essential for interpreting FNA cytology results, and the Bethesda System is commonly utilized for this purpose. This system classifies FNAB samples into six diagnostic categories, each associated with a specific estimated cancer risk:

- Non-diagnostic
- Benign
- Atypia/Follicular Lesion of Undetermined Significance (AUS/FLUS)
- Follicular Neoplasm
- Suspicious for Malignancy
- Malignant

Molecular Testing of FNAB Samples

Molecular testing of FNAB specimens for thyroid-specific genetic mutations can be valuable in further assessing thyroid nodules. Several commercial molecular panels are available to improve the accuracy of preoperative cytological diagnoses. After considering clinical and ultrasound characteristics, mutational analysis, such as testing for BRAF mutations or a seven-gene panel (including BRAF, RAS, RET/PTC, and PAX8/PPAR-Gamma), may be useful, particularly when cytology indicates suspicion of malignancy. These results can guide surgical decisions.

Laboratory Evaluation for Thyroid Nodules
A. Serum Thyroid-Stimulating Hormone (TSH)
Serum TSH should be measured using a highly sensitive immunometric assay in the initial evaluation of patients presenting with thyroid nodules or nontoxic goiters. If TSH levels are abnormal, free T4 (fT4) should also be assessed. A suppressed TSH may indicate the presence of toxic or autonomously functioning nodules, in which case thyroid scintigraphy is recommended. It is important to note that patients with thyroid cancer rarely exhibit abnormal TSH levels, whereas elevated TSH in patients with nontoxic goiters may suggest thyroiditis or hypothyroidism.

B. Serum Thyroid Autoantibodies

Testing for serum antithyroid peroxidase (TPO) antibodies or antithyroglobulin antibodies can aid in diagnosing chronic autoimmune thyroiditis. However, routine measurement of serum thyroglobulin is not recommended for the initial evaluation of thyroid nodules.

C. Serum Calcitonin

Serum calcitonin measurement is recommended for patients with a family history of medullary thyroid carcinoma (MTC) or when there is clinical suspicion of MTC or multiple endocrine neoplasia (MEN).

Serum Calcitonin and MEN2 Considerations

Measurement of serum calcitonin levels is recommended for individuals with a family history of medullary thyroid carcinoma (MTC) or when there is clinical suspicion of multiple endocrine neoplasia type 2 (MEN2). However, routine calcitonin testing in patients with thyroid nodules is neither cost-effective nor necessary unless there is a clinical suspicion of MTC or abnormal cytologic findings.

Additional Imaging Modalities for Thyroid Nodule and Goiter Evaluation

A. Radionuclide Scanning
Thyroid scintigraphy using technetium is advised for patients presenting with a solitary thyroid nodule or multi-nodular goiter accompanied by suppressed TSH levels.

B. CT and MRI
For patients with large goiters, conventional radiography of the neck and upper mediastinum should be utilized to evaluate any tracheal compression. CT and MRI are particularly beneficial for assessing invasion into adjacent structures or identifying retrosternal or intrathoracic goiters. These imaging modalities are also crucial in detecting occult metastases in the mediastinal and retropharyngeal areas during follow-up for patients post-thyroidectomy, especially in cases where serum thyroglobulin

(Tg) levels are elevated, but ultrasound findings are negative. CT and MRI can also provide access to difficult-to-evaluate nodal regions, such as the lower paratracheal nodes in the superior mediastinum (level VII) and the retropharyngeal and retroesophageal nodal groups, which are not easily visualized with ultrasound.

Management of Thyroid Nodules and Goiter

1. Observation and Monitoring
Patients with small, asymptomatic goiters may be managed through regular clinical examinations and periodic ultrasound evaluations. The growth patterns of goiters vary, and many patients experience minimal or no growth over several years.

2. Thyroid Hormone Suppression Therapy
Thyroid hormone suppression therapy has been shown to induce regression in cases of sporadic nontoxic diffuse goiters, as documented in earlier studies. However, nodular goiters and

thyroid nodules are less likely to respond to thyroxine suppression therapy for size reduction. Patients who are younger, have smaller nodules, or were recently diagnosed are more likely to benefit from this therapy. If treatment is discontinued, thyroid nodules typically return to their original size, necessitating ongoing therapy for sustained size reduction. However, prolonged thyroid hormone suppression therapy carries the risk of adverse effects, such as bone loss and cardiac tachyarrhythmias, particularly in older adults.

3. Surgery

Surgical intervention for nontoxic goiter may become necessary if the patient experiences progressive obstructive symptoms. In such cases, near-total or total thyroidectomy is typically the preferred procedure. However, if subtotal thyroidectomy is performed, there is a 10%–20% risk of recurrence within 10 years.

4. Radioiodine (131-I) Therapy

Radioiodine therapy (131-I) is a safe and effective treatment option for patients with nontoxic diffuse or multinodular goiters. Most patients experience a gradual reduction in goiter size following treatment. Initial side effects may include mild pain, tenderness, and transient thyrotoxicosis. In the long term, hypothyroidism can develop in up to 40% of patients receiving this therapy.

5. Alcohol Injection

Percutaneous ethanol injection is an option for treating recurrent symptomatic cystic nodules. This procedure can provide relief in selected cases.

Management Algorithm for Thyroid Nodules
Cytology Results (Bethesda System):
- Nondiagnostic:
  - Repeat FNA with ultrasound guidance and, if possible, on-site cytologic evaluation.
  - For repeatedly nondiagnostic nodules that do not exhibit a high-suspicion sonographic pattern,

close monitoring or surgical excision for histopathologic diagnosis is advised.

- Surgery should be considered if the nondiagnostic nodule shows a high-suspicion sonographic pattern, demonstrates growth (>20% in two dimensions) during ultrasound surveillance, or if there are clinical risk factors for malignancy.

For Nodules with AUS/FLUS, FN/FSN, or Suspicious Cytology

- AUS/FLUS Cytology: For nodules diagnosed with atypia of undetermined significance or follicular lesions of undetermined significance (AUS/FLUS), additional investigations such as repeat fine-needle aspiration (FNA) or molecular testing may be considered to refine the assessment of malignancy risk. This approach can help determine whether to proceed with surveillance or opt for diagnostic surgery. The decision should factor in patient preferences and the feasibility of each option.

- FN/SFN Cytology: In cases of follicular neoplasm or suspicious follicular neoplasm

(FN/SFN), diagnostic surgical excision may be appropriate. Alternatively, molecular testing can aid in malignancy risk stratification, potentially influencing the decision to forgo immediate surgery. As with AUS/FLUS, patient preference and the practicality of treatment options should guide clinical decision-making.

- Suspicious Cytology: When cytology indicates suspicion for papillary carcinoma, surgical management should align with the approach used for malignant cytology cases. Factors such as clinical risk, sonographic findings, patient preferences, and possible results from mutational testing should inform the treatment plan.

Chapter Five
Thyroid Emergencies and Perioperative Management of Thyroid Diseases

Thyroid Storm

Thyroid storm, a life-threatening form of thyrotoxicosis, is a rare but critical condition with an incidence of approximately 0.2 per 100,000 annually . This multisystem disorder carries a significant mortality risk, with rates ranging between 11% and 25% . It typically arises from a triggering event combined with underlying hyperthyroidism. Non-compliance with antithyroid medication is the leading precipitating factor, followed by severe infections, cardiac events, surgeries (thyroidal and non-thyroidal), trauma, iodinated contrast administration, radioactive iodine treatment, pregnancy, childbirth, adrenal insufficiency, and diabetic ketoacidosis .

The main cause of death in thyroid storms is multiorgan failure, particularly acute heart failure. Early recognition and aggressive treatment are crucial for improving patient outcomes. Given the high mortality rates, these patients should be managed in an intensive care unit (ICU) with a multidisciplinary team that includes endocrinologists, intensivists, cardiologists, hepatologists, and neurologists.

How Is Thyroid Storm Diagnosed?

Thyroid storm is diagnosed clinically in a patient with thyrotoxicosis who shows signs of decompensation. The diagnosis can be challenging due to overlapping symptoms with other critical illnesses. To improve diagnostic accuracy, objective methods such as the Burch–Wartofsky Point Scale (BWPS) and the Japan Thyroid Association (JTA) scoring system are utilized. These tools help distinguish thyroid storms from other severe medical conditions, enabling timely and effective treatment.

The BWPS (Burch-Wartofsky Point Scale) assesses patients by assigning scores based on various clinical criteria, including thermoregulatory disturbances, tachycardia/atrial fibrillation, congestive heart failure, central nervous system dysfunction, gastrointestinal and hepatic symptoms, as well as any precipitating events (refer to Table 9). A BWPS score of 45 or higher strongly suggests thyroid storm, a score between 25 and 44 indicates a risk of impending thyroid storm, and a score below 25 makes the diagnosis unlikely .

The Japan Thyroid Association (JTA) system takes a qualitative approach, categorizing patients into Thyroid Storm 1 (TS1) or Thyroid Storm 2 (TS2) based on the presence of thyrotoxicosis as a necessary condition (see Table 10) . Patients who meet the criteria for a BWPS score of 45 or above, or who are classified as JTA TS1 or TS2, and who show signs of decompensation, require prompt and aggressive multimodal treatment.

Burch–Wartofsky Criteria for Diagnosing Thyroid Storm

Thermoregulatory Dysfunction:
- Temperature:
  - 37.2–37.7°C (99–99.9°F): 5 points
  - 37.8–38.2°C (100–100.9°F): 10 points
  - 38.3–38.8°C (101–101.9°F): 15 points
  - 38.9–39.4°C (102–102.9°F): 20 points
  - 39.5–39.9°C (103–103.9°F): 25 points

Central Nervous System Effects:
- Absent: 0 points
- Mild (e.g., agitation): 10 points
- Moderate (e.g., delirium, psychosis, extreme lethargy): 20 points
- Severe (e.g., seizures, coma): 30 points

Gastrointestinal-Hepatic Dysfunction:
- Absent: 0 points
- Moderate (e.g., diarrhea, nausea/vomiting, abdominal pain): 10 points
- Severe (e.g., unexplained jaundice): 20 points

Cardiovascular Dysfunction:
- Tachycardia:

- 90–109 bpm: 5 points
   - 110–119 bpm: 10 points
   - 120–129 bpm: 15 points
   - 130–139 bpm: 20 points
   - ≥140 bpm: 25 points
- Congestive Heart Failure:
   - Absent: 0 points
   - Mild (e.g., pedal edema): 5 points
   - Moderate (e.g., bibasilar rales): 10 points
   - Severe (e.g., pulmonary edema): 15 points
- Atrial Fibrillation:
   - Absent: 0 points
   - Present: 10 points

Precipitating History:
- Negative: 0 points
- Positive: 10 points

Interpretation:
- A total score of ≥45 strongly suggests thyroid storm.
- A score of 25–44 indicates a possible impending storm.

- A score below 25 makes a thyroid storm unlikely.

(Adapted from Burch–Wartofsky Point Scale (BWPS), Level III)

In cases of severe thyrotoxicosis, the highest applicable score in each category should be used. If it's difficult to differentiate between effects of an intercurrent illness and those of thyrotoxicosis, points should be assigned to support the diagnosis of a storm to ensure timely empirical treatment.

Japan Thyroid Association Diagnostic Criteria for Thyroid Storm

Prerequisite for Diagnosis:
Presence of thyrotoxicosis, characterized by elevated levels of free triiodothyronine (FT3) or free thyroxinc (FT4).

Symptoms:

1. Central Nervous System (CNS) Manifestations:

Restlessness, delirium, mental disturbances/psychosis, drowsiness/lethargy, or coma

(≥1 on the Japan Coma Scale or ≤14 on the Glasgow Coma Scale).

2. Fever:

Temperature of ≥38°C.

3. Tachycardia:

Heart rate ≥130 beats per minute, or ≥130 in patients with atrial fibrillation.

4. Congestive Heart Failure (CHF):

Symptoms include pulmonary edema, moist rales over more than half of the lung field, cardiogenic shock,

or New York Heart Association (NYHA) Class IV or Killip Classification ≥Class III.

5. Gastrointestinal (GI)/Hepatic Manifestations:

Symptoms include nausea, vomiting, diarrhea, or a total bilirubin level of ≥3.0 mg/dL.

(Adapted from Japan Thyroid Association, Level III)

Diagnosis:

Grade of Thyroid Storm (TS)	Combination of Features	Diagnostic Requirements
TS1	**Primary Combination:**	Thyrotoxicosis and at least one CNS manifestation, plus fever, tachycardia, CHF, or GI/hepatic manifestations.
TS1A	**Alternate Combination:**	Thyrotoxicosis and at least three of the

		following: fever, tachycardia, CHF, or GI/hepatic manifestations.
TS2	**Primary Combination:**	Thyrotoxicosis and two of the following: fever, tachycardia, CHF, or GI/hepatic manifestations.
TS2	**Alternate Combination:**	Meets the criteria for TS1, but serum FT3 or FT4 levels are unavailable

Exclusion and Provisions:

Cases should be excluded if symptoms such as fever, impaired consciousness, heart failure, or liver dysfunction are clearly due to other underlying conditions (e.g., pneumonia, malignant hyperthermia, psychiatric disorders, cerebrovascular disease, acute myocardial infarction, viral hepatitis, or acute liver failure). In situations where it is difficult to distinguish between thyroid storm and symptoms of other diseases, the symptoms should be considered as being due to thyroid storm precipitated by these factors. Clinical judgment is essential in making this determination.

TS1: Definite thyroid storm
TS2: Suspected thyroid storm

Treatment Considerations

The choice of aggressive treatment for patients with a Burch-Wartofsky Point Scale (BWPS) score of 25–44 should be based on clinical judgment, balancing the risks of treatment-related adverse events. Retrospective analyses show that both the BWPS and Japan Thyroid Association (JTA) diagnostic tools generally align, though the JTA may under-diagnose thyroid storms. If there is uncertainty about whether symptoms are caused by thyroid storm or another condition, it is prudent to treat as if thyroid storm is present. Although measurements of free T4 (fT4), free T3 (fT3), and thyroid-stimulating hormone (TSH) are necessary, they may not reflect the clinical severity.

Recommendations:
- Diagnosis of thyroid storm is primarily clinical. Both the BWPS and JTA diagnostic tools can assist, but the BWPS is preferred due to its higher sensitivity.
- A BWPS score of ≥45 or JTA TS1 confirms thyroid storm.

- A BWPS score of 25–44 or JTA TS2 requires clinical judgment to assess for decompensation and confirm the diagnosis of thyroid storm.

Anti-Thyroid Drug Choice in Thyroid Storm

Early and intensive treatment is crucial for managing thyroid storms. The therapeutic approach focuses on:

a) Inhibiting thyroid hormone synthesis and release
b) Counteracting the peripheral effects of thyroid hormones
c) Addressing systemic decompensation
d) Treating the underlying precipitating event
e) Implementing definitive therapy

High doses of propylthiouracil (PTU) or methimazole (MMI) are used to inhibit thyroid hormone synthesis and release. Recommended dosing is 500–1000 mg for PTU, followed by 250 mg every four hours, and 60–80 mg/day for MMI, either as a single dose or in two divided doses. PTU is generally preferred in thyroid storms because it inhibits type I deiodinase activity, reducing T4 conversion to T3, with T3 levels decreasing by approximately 45% within one hour of PTU administration compared to 10%–15% with MMI. However, a nationwide survey in Japan found no significant difference in outcomes between PTU and MMI treatments.

MMI has the advantages of less frequent dosing and reduced hepatotoxicity. Given the high doses of antithyroid drugs administered, monitoring for adverse effects such as liver dysfunction, rash, and agranulocytosis is essential.

Recommendations

- High-Dose Antithyroid Medications: In cases of thyroid storm, high doses of propylthiouracil (PTU) are recommended, typically starting with 500–1000 mg as a loading dose followed by 250 mg every 4–6 hours. If PTU is contraindicated, methimazole (MMI) at 60–80 mg per day can be used. Once the thyroid storm condition improves, patients should be transitioned to MMI.

- Rectal Antithyroid Drugs: When oral administration of PTU or MMI is not feasible, such as in patients with impaired gastrointestinal absorption or those on mechanical ventilation, rectal formulations can be utilized. The dosage and frequency of rectal PTU or MMI are similar to their oral counterparts. Rectal PTU has been shown to be effective in managing thyroid storms.

 - Rectal PTU Preparation:
    - PTU enema: 400 mg of PTU in 90 mL of sterile water.
     - PTU suppository: 200 mg of PTU in a polyethylene glycol base.

- Beta-Adrenergic Receptor Antagonists: Beta-blockers play a crucial role in managing thyroid storms by controlling heart rate and counteracting the peripheral effects of thyroid hormones. Propranolol, a non-selective beta-blocker, is preferred due to its ability to inhibit type 1 deiodinase, with a typical dose of 60–80 mg every four hours. In patients with significant cardiac compromise or decompensated heart failure, selective beta-1 blockers such as bisoprolol, landiolol, and esmolol are more suitable. If beta-blockers are contraindicated, cardioselective calcium-channel blockers like diltiazem or intravenous esmolol can be used in the intensive care setting to manage heart rate.

- Intravenous Esmolol Administration:
  - Loading dose: 250–500 mcg/kg
  - Maintenance infusion: 50–100 mcg/kg/min, adjusted based on heart rate and blood pressure.

- Cardioversion and Anticoagulation: In cases of atrial fibrillation, cardioversion should be considered if hemodynamics are compromised and after excluding cardiac thrombosis. Anticoagulation may be required if the CHADS2 score is ≥2.

Recommendations

- Beta-Adrenergic Receptor Antagonists: Use beta-adrenergic blockers such as propranolol to manage heart rate and mitigate the peripheral effects of thyroid hormones during a thyroid storm. If beta-blockers are contraindicated, alternative treatments like intravenous esmolol or diltiazem should be considered for heart rate control.

- Corticosteroids: Administer high doses of corticosteroids in thyroid storm to inhibit thyroid hormone synthesis and the conversion of T4 to T3, and to provide prophylaxis against adrenal insufficiency due to the hypermetabolic state. Recommended options include intravenous hydrocortisone (100 mg every 6 hours) or dexamethasone (2 mg every 6 hours). Dosages should be reduced and tapered as the patient's condition improves to minimize adverse effects.

- Inorganic Iodide: Use inorganic iodide solutions, such as Lugol's iodine or saturated solution of potassium iodide (SSKI), to rapidly lower T4 levels by inhibiting iodide oxidation, organification, and hormone release. Administer 5 drops of Lugol's iodine every 6 hours (6.25 mg iodine per drop) or 10 drops every 8 hours. Ensure iodide is given at least one hour after antithyroid drugs to avoid interference with thyroid hormone synthesis. Discontinue Lugol's iodine after clinical improvement and do not use it beyond 10 days to avoid the Wolff-Chaikoff effect. If necessary, inorganic iodide can be given rectally or via nasogastric tube in critically ill patients, with solutions diluted in water or taken with bread to prevent mucosal irritation.

Recommendations

- Lugol's Iodine: Administer 5–10 drops of Lugol's iodine every 6–8 hours for up to 10 days to achieve rapid improvement in thyrotoxicosis during thyroid storm. This treatment should follow the administration of antithyroid medications.

- Lithium and Cholecystographic Agents: Lithium can be used as an alternative treatment for patients who cannot tolerate methimazole (MMI) or propylthiouracil (PTU), working by an unknown mechanism to inhibit thyroid hormone release. The recommended dose is 300 mg up to three times daily, with close monitoring to avoid toxicity and nephrogenic diabetes insipidus. Cholestyramine can also be employed to reduce thyrotoxicosis by decreasing enterohepatic recycling of thyroid hormones. The recommended dose is 1–4 grams every 6 hours.

- Plasma Exchange: Total plasma exchange (TPE) is indicated for severe thyroid storms, especially when there is rapid deterioration or failure of standard therapy. TPE is effective in removing thyroid hormones, antibodies, and cytokines, and is recommended with 40–50 mL/kg of replacement fluid. Plasma exchange should be continued until clinical improvement is observed, with fT4 and fT3 levels monitored before and after each session. Fresh frozen plasma (FFP) is preferred over albumin due to its thyroid-binding globulin content, which enhances the removal of bound thyroid hormones. Continuous hemodiafiltration (CHDF) may be used in conjunction with TPE in patients with significant hemodynamic instability.

Role of Supportive Therapy

In the management of thyroid storm, supportive therapies are essential. These therapies include administering intravenous fluids, providing respiratory support, and ensuring adequate nutritional support. Cooling measures, such as using cooling blankets and administering acetaminophen, are recommended. Salicylates should be avoided as they can displace bound thyroxine, potentially increasing free thyroid hormone levels. Broad-spectrum antibiotics should be used to address infections, with selection tailored to the infection source. In cases of respiratory failure or severe central nervous system depression, both invasive and non-invasive ventilation may be necessary.

Recommendation:

- Avoid salicylates, as they displace bound thyroxine, leading to elevated levels of free thyroid hormone.

Role of Early Definitive Therapy and Prevention

Definitive therapy should be considered for all patients with thyroid storm. In cases where antithyroid drugs are contraindicated or in the presence of a large goiter, urgent thyroidectomy may be necessary. Patients should ideally be brought close to a euthyroid state prior to surgery, potentially using methods such as therapeutic plasma exchange (TPE), to minimize the risk of exacerbating thyroid storm. If radioactive iodine (RAI) therapy is planned, it should be delayed 3-4 months if Lugol's iodine has been administered during the storm. Education on the importance of adherence is crucial, as non-compliance is a common precipitating factor. Patients scheduled for surgery or RAI should be as near euthyroid as possible before proceeding or consider postponing the procedure to prevent thyroid storm.

Recommendation:
- All patients with thyroid storm should receive early definitive therapy with RAI. For patients with large obstructing goiters, early thyroidectomy should be considered.

Myxoedema Coma

Diagnosis of Myxoedema Coma

Myxoedema coma is a rare but serious condition diagnosed primarily through clinical presentation, including reduced consciousness and hypothermia. Thyroid function tests will typically indicate hypothyroidism. Additional clinical signs may include hyponatremia and/or hypercapnia. The diagnosis should be considered in patients with a history of hypothyroidism or any underlying cause of hypothyroidism. It is important to rule out other potential causes of decreased consciousness.

Diagnostic Scoring Systems for Myxoedema Coma

Diagnostic scoring systems have been developed but lack robust validation due to the low incidence of myxoedema coma. (Level III)

Complications of Myxoedema Coma

Myxoedema coma is a severe systemic condition that can impact multiple organ systems. Recognized complications include:

- Metabolic: Hypoglycemia, hyponatremia
- Cardiovascular: Bradycardia, hypotension, pericardial effusion, heart failure
- Neurological: Psychosis, seizures, altered consciousness
- Respiratory: Hypoventilation, hypercapnia, sleep apnea

- Renal: Failure
- Hematological: Anemia
(Level III)

Optimal Treatment Modalities for Myxoedema Coma

Patients with myxoedema coma require intensive care. Due to potential impairment in oral medication absorption, intravenous thyroxine is generally preferred. Intravenous hydrocortisone is also recommended, particularly if there is concurrent hypoadrenalism, with a serum cortisol level ideally measured before administration.

Recommendations:
- Administer intravenous hydrocortisone 200 mg stat, followed by 100 mg every 6–8 hours prior to initiating levothyroxine.
- Begin with an intravenous dose of levothyroxine 200–400 mcg, then maintain at 1.6 mcg/kg/day (75% if administered intravenously). If intravenous levothyroxine is

unavailable, initiate oral levothyroxine with a 500 mcg loading dose, followed by a maintenance dose.

- If available, intravenous liothyronine may be added to levothyroxine therapy, starting with 5–20 mcg as a loading dose, followed by 2.5–10 mcg every 8 hours until the patient regains consciousness.

(Level II, III)

Monitoring of Patients with Myxoedema Coma

Patients should show signs of improvement within one week of treatment. Continuous monitoring of multiple organ systems is essential, including mental status, cardiovascular function, respiratory parameters, renal function, and metabolic status (e.g., electrolytes). Thyroid function tests should be performed every two days. The Sequential Organ Failure Assessment (SOFA) score is a useful tool for evaluating patient outcomes, demonstrating higher predictive value compared to other assessment tools.

(Level II, III)

Pre-/Perioperative Management: Hyperthyroidism

Surgical stress and anesthesia may trigger thyroid storm, cardiac failure, or tachyarrhythmias in patients with uncontrolled hyperthyroidism. However, morbidity and mortality rates are generally low in patients who are well-prepared. (Level III)

Optimal Treatment and Risk Minimization

A combination of antithyroid medications, beta-blockers, iodine, and glucocorticoids has been effective in quickly controlling hyperthyroidism in surgical patients. Studies suggest that beta-blockade alone may lead to better perioperative outcomes compared to antithyroid drugs alone. (Level II, III)

Recommendations:

- Elective surgeries should be deferred until the patient achieves a euthyroid or near-euthyroid state.
- For urgent surgeries, assess the patient's thyroid status both clinically and biochemically.
- In hyperthyroid patients requiring urgent surgery, rapid control with high-dose methimazole (MMI) or propylthiouracil (PTU), beta-blockers, Lugol's iodine, and glucocorticoids is recommended. (Level II, III)

Preoperative Treatment for Subclinical Hyperthyroidism

Recommendations:
- Treatment is generally advised only for elderly patients and those with pre-existing cardiac conditions or atrial fibrillation who have subclinical hyperthyroidism.
- Beta-blockers should be used to reduce the risk of tachyarrhythmias during the perioperative period in elderly patients and those with pre-existing cardiac conditions and subclinical hyperthyroidism.

Preoperative Management: Hypothyroidism

Universal Screening for Hypothyroidism

There is insufficient evidence to support or refute the practice of universal screening for hypothyroidism before surgery. Expert opinions vary regarding which subpopulations should be screened. (Level II)

Recommendations:

- Universal screening for hypothyroidism before surgery is not recommended.
- Screening should be conducted only for patients with risk factors for hypothyroidism or those showing symptoms.

Potential Intraoperative and Postoperative Complications of Untreated Hypothyroidism

Untreated hypothyroidism results in systemic hypometabolism and can lead to several complications, including hypotension, cardiovascular collapse, hypoventilation, heightened sensitivity to opioids, sedatives, and anesthesia, and myxedema coma. Patients with overt hypothyroidism face a higher risk of cardiovascular issues, and similar risks are noted in those with mild hypothyroidism. Subclinical hypothyroidism is also linked with obstructive sleep apnea, which can impact intubation and ventilation. (Level II)

Management of Perioperative Hypothyroidism

Postoperative outcomes vary with the severity of hypothyroidism. Mild (subclinical) and moderate (overt) hypothyroidism typically present fewer complications. However, severe hypothyroidism (myxedema coma) poses a higher surgical risk.

Recommendations:
- For mild hypothyroidism (subclinical), surgery can proceed as scheduled.
- For moderate hypothyroidism (overt), urgent surgeries can be performed without delay, but

elective surgeries should ideally wait until the patient achieves a euthyroid state.

- For severe hypothyroidism (myxedema coma), both T3 and T4 treatment should be administered before surgery.

Chapter Six
Thyroiditis – Subacute and Acute Thyroiditis

Subacute Thyroiditis (De Quervain's Thyroiditis)

Diagnosis of Subacute Thyroiditis

Subacute thyroiditis is a cause of thyroid gland pain, typically presenting between the ages of 40 and 50. It shows a higher prevalence in females, with a significant gender ratio noted in various studies.

Subacute Thyroiditis (De Quervain's Thyroiditis)

Diagnosis of Subacute Thyroiditis

Subacute thyroiditis is characterized by painful thyroid swelling, which is a key diagnostic indicator. Prodromal symptoms, such as upper respiratory tract symptoms, are reported in varying frequencies, with some studies indicating their presence in 20% to 38.5% of cases. Fever is observed in 12.5% to 46.2% of patients.

Typically, subacute thyroiditis presents during the thyrotoxic phase, which begins 1 to 2 weeks after onset. Hyperthyroidism generally lasts for 2 to 3 weeks, peaking around 1 week after onset, followed by a hypothyroid phase lasting 6 to 12 weeks before returning to a euthyroid state. Most studies show a moderate increase in thyroxine levels with suppressed thyroid-stimulating hormone (TSH), while thyroid storm is rare. The free triiodothyronine (fT3) to free thyroxine (fT4) ratio is notably lower in subacute thyroiditis compared to Graves' disease, with an fT3/fT4 ratio below 0.3 showing 52.4% sensitivity and 91.3% specificity for destructive thyroiditis. Thyroglobulin levels are elevated in subacute thyroiditis, and thyroid antibodies are present in 4% to 20% of cases, although their titre is generally lower compared to Graves' disease.

An elevated erythrocyte sedimentation rate (ESR) is a significant diagnostic marker, with average levels around 60 mm in the first hour, though some studies report levels as high as 100 mm. C-reactive protein (CRP) levels are also elevated in this condition. Imaging often reveals low uptake on radio-iodine scans, and while neck ultrasound may show ill-defined hypoechoic lesions, Doppler ultrasound indicating suppressed vascularity can be useful. A study found that 77.8% of patients had hypoechoic lesions, and 95% had reduced Doppler color flow. Another study described a "lava flow" appearance on grayscale ultrasound in all cases examined.

Recommendations:
- Subacute thyroiditis should be considered in all patients presenting with a painful goiter.

Within six weeks, the majority of patients recover from subacute thyroiditis, though 30% require seven to eight weeks, and 20% take more than eight weeks for complete recovery. A Level II retrospective study indicates that tapering prednisolone from 30 mg to 5 mg daily over an extended period (up to 44 days) correlates with a lack of recurrence (Level III evidence).

An experimental approach involves injecting a combination of lidocaine and dexamethasone directly into the thyroid gland using an insulin pen. Although the prospective study yielded seemingly favorable outcomes, with a small sample size of 36 participants, further research is needed to clarify its efficacy and safety (Level III evidence).

Recommendation:
- Prednisolone Tapering: A recommended regimen starts with 15 mg/day, gradually reducing to 5 mg/day every two weeks. Prolonged prednisolone use may be necessary for patients with persistent symptoms or elevated ESR or CRP levels.

Follow-up Duration for Subacute Thyroiditis:

Retrospective studies suggest that long-term recurrence of subacute thyroiditis is very rare. One study (Level III evidence) reported a recurrence rate of only 1.6% over a 13-year period. However, recurrence rates are higher within the first year, and they decline over time. Another retrospective study (Level III evidence) observed a recurrence rate of approximately 10% over five years of follow-up, with a 10% recurrence within the first year and 4% after one year. Hypothyroidism rates were reported at 34% in the first year and 15% after one year (Level III evidence). Therefore, frequent follow-up within the first year is advisable, with progressively less frequent follow-ups over the next five years. After five years, follow-up may not be necessary.

Recommendation:
- Monitoring: Patients should undergo follow-up every six months during the first year and annually for the subsequent five years.

Diagnosis of Acute (Suppurative) Thyroiditis:

Acute thyroiditis is a rare but potentially life-threatening condition. Its clinical presentation is similar to subacute thyroiditis but with greater severity. Prominent symptoms include significant pain, fever, and lymphadenopathy. Inflammation from the condition may lead to upper airway obstruction, and patients often adopt a posture that limits neck extension. The presence of fluctuance suggests the development of an abscess (Level I evidence).

Acute thyroiditis typically presents with a euthyroid state, but there are case reports of patients experiencing hyperthyroidism and even thyroid storm (Level III evidence). During the early inflammatory phase, ultrasound may not detect a well-defined hypoechoic lesion; instead, it often shows a diffuse hypoechoic area throughout the thyroid lobe, which could lead to a misdiagnosis of subacute thyroiditis (Level III evidence). Approximately one week later, a thyroid abscess or a clearly demarcated hypoechoic lesion usually becomes evident.

Other imaging techniques, such as CT scans and MRIs, are also useful in identifying abscesses (Level III evidence).

Moreover, identifying a pyriform sinus fistula is critical, as it can contribute to recurrence. This fistula can be detected through direct endoscopy, barium esophagography, or CT scan (Level III evidence).

Recommendations:
- Clinical Suspicion: Acute thyroiditis should be suspected in any patient presenting with a painful goiter.
- Diagnostic Testing: All patients with painful thyroid swelling should undergo thyroid function tests, including free thyroxine and thyroid-stimulating hormone levels.
- Imaging: An ultrasound should be performed in all patients with painful thyroid swelling to exclude acute or suppurative thyroiditis. If the initial ultrasound is non-diagnostic within the first week of symptom onset, it should be repeated later.

- Aspiration and Culture: If the ultrasound suggests an abscess or acute/suppurative thyroiditis, aspiration should be performed, and the sample sent for Gram stain, culture, and sensitivity testing.
- Immunocompromised Patients: In immunocompromised individuals with atypical presentations, rare causative organisms, such as tuberculosis, should be considered.

Management of Acute Thyroiditis:

Fine needle aspiration of the thyroid, followed by Gram staining, culture, and sensitivity testing, is essential to identify the causative organism. Commonly reported bacterial isolates include Streptococcus pyogenes, Staphylococcus aureus, and Streptococcus pneumoniae (Level III evidence). Additionally, Gram-negative bacteria such as Haemophilus influenzae, Escherichia coli, and Klebsiella species have been documented (Level III evidence). Therefore, empirical broad-spectrum antibiotics are appropriate for initial management. Less than

1% of cases involve tuberculosis as the causative agent (Level III evidence).

The primary treatment for acute thyroiditis is surgical excision (Level III evidence). To prevent recurrence, the pyriform sinus fistula may be surgically removed or chemically obliterated, with favorable outcomes reported in case series (Level III evidence). With prompt and effective antibiotic therapy and the removal of any abscesses, patients generally have an excellent prognosis if they survive the acute phase.

The low incidence of acute thyroiditis makes it difficult to determine the exact morbidity and mortality rates associated with the condition. However, with proper treatment, the prognosis is generally good.

Recommendations:
- Symptomatic Management: Beta-blockers may be used in patients experiencing symptoms of thyrotoxicosis.

- Treatment Strategy: Acute or suppurative thyroiditis should be managed with antibiotics, and surgical drainage should be considered based on clinical judgment.

Chapter Seven
Special Considerations

Hypothyroidism and Pregnancy
Definition of Maternal Overt and Subclinical Hypothyroidism (OH/SCHypo)

Maternal hypothyroidism is typically defined by an elevated serum TSH level during pregnancy that exceeds the upper limit of the pregnancy-specific reference range. Overt hypothyroidism is also marked by a low serum free T4 (fT4) level below the pregnancy-specific reference range, while subclinical hypothyroidism (SCHypo) is indicated by an elevated TSH with a normal fT4 level. Currently, serum TSH is the primary indicator used to guide treatment and target levels. However, there are significant variations in the upper reference limit of pregnancy-specific TSH ranges between different populations, ranging from 2.15 to 4.68 mIU/L (Level II evidence).

It is, therefore, recommended that each institution establish its own pregnancy-specific reference intervals for each trimester, based on the local population. If specific local data is unavailable, a TSH upper limit of 4 mIU/L can be used. This figure represents a reduction of 0.5 mIU/L from the non-pregnant TSH upper limit in most assays (Level II evidence).

Recommendations:
- Institution-Specific Guidelines: Each institution should establish its own pregnancy-specific reference intervals for each trimester, based on the local population.
- Interim Standard for Malaysia: In the absence of published data for the Malaysian pregnant population, a TSH upper reference limit of 4 mIU/L is recommended.

Prevalence and Common Causes of Maternal Hypothyroidism

The prevalence of hypothyroidism during pregnancy ranges from 0.3% to 4.8% (Level II and III evidence). The onset of hypothyroidism during pregnancy is rare (Level II evidence). The most common cause of hypothyroidism in pregnancy is chronic autoimmune thyroiditis (Hashimoto's thyroiditis) (Level III evidence). Other causes may include prior thyroid surgery or radiation therapy.

Other causes of hypothyroidism in pregnancy include prior thyroid surgery, radioiodine ablation, congenital hypothyroidism, and less commonly, lymphocytic hypophysitis (Level III evidence). Additionally, a high pre-pregnancy body mass index (BMI) is a notable risk factor for developing hypothyroidism during pregnancy.

A retrospective cohort study indicated an elevated risk of miscarriage in pregnant women who were treated with LT4 before conception and had a TSH level above 2.5 mIU/L in the first trimester (Level II evidence). Currently, no clinical studies have been conducted to determine the optimal TSH level in the second or third trimester. However, similar to the management of hypothyroidism in the general population, it is reasonable to target TSH levels in the lower half of the trimester-specific reference range for the local population (Level II evidence). In the absence of local pregnancy-specific reference ranges, a preconception and first-trimester TSH target of ≤2.5 mIU/L is recommended. This target can be relaxed to 3.0 mIU/L during the second and third trimesters (Level III evidence). After delivery, the TSH goal can return to the normal non-pregnant reference range, as long as the patient is not planning another immediate pregnancy.

Recommendations:
- TSH Target for Hypothyroid Women on LT4: For women already receiving LT4 before conception, a target TSH level of ≤2.5 mIU/L is recommended both before conception and during the first trimester, given the lack of trimester-specific reference ranges for the Malaysian population.

Recommendations:
- TSH Goal for Second and Third Trimester: During the second and third trimesters, a TSH target of 3.0 mIU/L or below is recommended.
- Postpartum TSH Goal: After delivery, TSH levels can be adjusted to the normal reference range for non-pregnant women.

Levothyroxine Requirements During Pregnancy and Postpartum: Monitoring Guidelines

Levothyroxine (LT4) requirements typically begin to increase as early as 4 to 6 weeks of gestation. The demand continues to rise until around 16–20 weeks (mid-gestation) and stabilizes throughout the third trimester until delivery (Level II evidence).

A retrospective observational study reported a 45%–70% increase in LT4 dosage by the end of pregnancy for women already on LT4 prior to conception (Level II evidence). Another study highlighted an LT4 dose increase of 13%–27% during the first trimester, which escalated to 26%–51% in the second trimester, with no significant rise during the third trimester (Level II evidence). The dose increase is generally higher in women with hypothyroidism caused by thyroidectomy or radioactive iodine treatment compared to those with autoimmune thyroiditis (Level II evidence).

A randomized controlled trial (RCT) comparing two strategies for LT4 dose adjustment in early pregnancy—either increasing by two tablets per week (29%) or three tablets per week (43%)—found both strategies effective in maintaining target TSH levels. However, the two-tablet strategy was associated with a lower risk of overtreatment and TSH suppression (Level I evidence). This study used a target TSH of up to 4.9 mIU/L, which exceeds the pregnancy-specific TSH upper limit for most populations (Level II evidence). Additionally, four-week thyroid function testing intervals were shown to identify over 90% of abnormal values during pregnancy (Level I evidence).

Given that the increased LT4 requirement during pregnancy is driven by the physiological need for a larger total thyroxine pool, the LT4 dosage should generally be reduced to pre-pregnancy levels after delivery. However, an observational study found that women with Hashimoto's thyroiditis might require a higher LT4 dose postpartum compared to pre-conception, possibly due to a postpartum flare of autoimmune thyroiditis (Level II evidence).

Recommendations:
- LT4 Dose Adjustment Upon Conception: For pregnant women on LT4 prior to conception, it is recommended to increase the LT4 dose by 30%–50% upon conception, with a higher percentage considered for those with post-ablative hypothyroidism and a lower percentage for autoimmune hypothyroidism.
- Thyroid Function Monitoring: Thyroid function should be tested every four weeks from conception until mid-gestation and at least once during the middle of the third trimester.

- Postpartum LT4 Adjustment: After delivery, the LT4 dosage should generally be adjusted back to the pre-pregnancy level.

Who Should Be Screened for Maternal Hypothyroidism?

Although untreated maternal hypothyroidism is linked to adverse pregnancy outcomes, universal screening for hypothyroidism during pregnancy remains a subject of debate. A prospective randomized controlled trial (RCT) comparing universal screening with a targeted case-finding approach showed no significant difference in adverse outcomes between the two methods (Level I evidence). As a result, the case-finding approach is recommended over universal screening for detecting maternal hypothyroidism.

The preferred test for screening is thyroid-stimulating hormone (TSH), as it is the most sensitive indicator of hypothyroidism. Risk factors associated with an increased likelihood of maternal hypothyroidism include a personal history of thyroid dysfunction, the presence of a goiter, known thyroid antibody positivity, age 30 years or older, type 1 diabetes or other autoimmune disorders, a history of pregnancy loss or preterm delivery, infertility, previous thyroid surgery or head and neck radiation, morbid obesity, use of lithium or amiodarone, recent use of iodinated contrast agents, residence in regions with moderate to severe iodine deficiency, family history of thyroid disorders, and having had two or more previous pregnancies (Level II evidence).

Hyperthyroidism and Pregnancy

Prevalence of Hyperthyroidism in Pregnancy

Globally, the prevalence of hyperthyroidism in pregnancy varies between 0.1% and 1.6% (Level II and III evidence). In the United States, two studies have reported incidence rates of 5.9 per 1,000 women and 3.77 per 1,000 women, respectively (Level II and III evidence). In Malaysia, studies have shown an incidence of 0.9 per 1,000 deliveries (Level II evidence). The onset of hyperthyroidism during pregnancy is rare, with Graves' disease being the most common cause (Level III and II evidence). A personal history of thyroid disorders or a family history of thyroid dysfunction has been associated with an increased risk of hyperthyroidism (Level II evidence)

Definition of Maternal Hyperthyroidism

Maternal hyperthyroidism is characterized by suppressed serum TSH levels accompanied by elevated free triiodothyronine (fT3) and/or free thyroxine (fT4). Subclinical hyperthyroidism, on the other hand, is defined as suppressed serum TSH levels with normal fT4 and/or fT3 levels. Notably, subclinical hyperthyroidism in pregnant women has not been linked to adverse maternal or fetal outcomes, and treatment for this condition is generally not recommended (Level III evidence). During the first trimester of a normal pregnancy, TSH levels naturally decline as a physiological response to the stimulating effect of human chorionic gonadotropin (hCG) on the TSH receptor, with peak hCG levels occurring during this period.

During weeks 7 to 11 of gestation, TSH levels decrease as part of a normal pregnancy. However, reference ranges for TSH and free thyroxine (fT4) can differ across populations due to variations in assays, ethnicity, and body mass index (BMI). The lower reference limit for pregnancy-specific TSH levels ranges from 0.02 to 0.41 mIU/L across different populations (Level II evidence). Therefore, any subnormal TSH level should be interpreted alongside serum fT4 levels. It is recommended that institutions establish trimester-specific reference ranges for TSH and fT4 based on local population data (Level II evidence).

Recommendations:
- Each healthcare institution should develop its own pregnancy-specific reference intervals for

each trimester using data from the local population.

- If serum TSH is found to be suppressed during the first trimester, a thorough medical history, physical examination, and maternal serum fT4 testing should be conducted.

Common Causes of Hyperthyroidism in Pregnancy

The primary causes of hyperthyroidism during pregnancy are gestational transient thyrotoxicosis (GTT) and Graves' disease (Level III evidence). Other causes include toxic multinodular goiter, toxic adenoma, and thyroiditis (Level III evidence). Rarely, hyperthyroidism in pregnancy may be caused by elevated beta-HCG levels, which can occur in cases of multiple gestation, molar pregnancy, or choriocarcinoma. These cases are often subclinical (Level III evidence).

Differentiating Gestational Transient Thyrotoxicosis (GTT) from Graves' Disease (GD)

Gestational transient thyrotoxicosis (GTT) is a non-autoimmune condition that usually occurs in the first trimester. It is triggered by elevated human chorionic gonadotropin (hCG) levels during early pregnancy, resulting in biochemical hyperthyroidism (Level III evidence). GTT is generally mild, asymptomatic, and self-limiting, though more severe cases may be associated with hyperemesis, leading to symptoms of hyperthyroidism (Level III evidence).

In early pregnancy, differentiating GTT from Graves' disease is essential since both conditions can cause elevated T4 levels and suppressed TSH levels (Level III evidence). Although the clinical presentations, such as palpitations, anxiety, tremors, and heat intolerance, may be similar, a careful review of the patient's medical history and a thorough physical examination are crucial in determining the cause (Level III evidence).

Patients without a history of thyroid disease, Graves' disease stigmata (e.g., goiter or ophthalmopathy), or TSH-receptor antibodies (TRAb) are more likely to have GTT (Level III evidence). The presence of TRAb is a strong indicator of Graves' disease, while anti-thyroid peroxidase antibodies (anti-TPO) can be found in both conditions (Level III evidence). Currently, there is no evidence to support the utility of thyroid testing for these conditions.

Ultrasound has limited value in distinguishing between gestational transient thyrotoxicosis (GTT) and Graves' disease (GD) (Level III evidence). Similarly, beta-hCG levels have restricted clinical utility in differentiating between these two conditions (Level II evidence).

Recommendation:

- When suppressed TSH and elevated fT4 levels are identified in the first trimester, a thorough clinical history and physical examination should be conducted to determine the underlying cause. Graves' disease can be differentiated from GTT based on clinical presentation, with TRAb supporting the diagnosis of Graves' disease.

Management of Gestational Transient Thyrotoxicosis (GTT)

Gestational transient thyrotoxicosis (GTT) is generally not associated with negative pregnancy outcomes (Level II evidence). Management is typically focused on symptom control, depending on the severity of the symptoms (Level III evidence). In cases of hyperemesis gravidarum, treatment with antiemetics and intravenous fluids is recommended, and hospitalization may be necessary in some instances. Antithyroid drugs (ATDs) are not recommended because they do not improve obstetric outcomes and carry an increased risk of birth defects when used in early pregnancy

(Level II evidence). However, no studies have compared the efficacy of ATDs to supportive therapy (Level III evidence). For patients with significant symptoms, short-term use of low-dose beta-blockers may be considered (Level III evidence). Serum T4 levels generally normalize between 14 and 18 weeks of gestation.

Recommendation:
- Management of GTT should primarily involve supportive care, including rehydration and hospitalization if necessary for hyperemesis gravidarum. Beta-blockers may be used for severe symptoms. Antithyroid drugs are not recommended.

Complications of Hyperthyroidism in Pregnancy

Uncontrolled hyperthyroidism during pregnancy can result in significant maternal and fetal complications (Level II evidence). Maternal complications include miscarriage, preterm delivery, hypertension, heart failure, and thyroid storm (Level III evidence). Additionally, transplacental transfer of TRAb antibodies can stimulate the fetal thyroid gland, potentially leading to fetal hyperthyroidism, which can cause intrauterine growth retardation, stillbirth, and low birth weight (Level II evidence). Conversely, fetal hypothyroidism may occur if the mother is treated with antithyroid drugs, particularly if the mother achieves a euthyroid state (Level III evidence).

Management of Graves' Disease Before Conception

Given that both hyperthyroidism and its treatments can lead to pregnancy complications, preconception counseling is essential for women of reproductive age with hyperthyroidism. Counseling should emphasize the importance of achieving a stable euthyroid state before attempting pregnancy, as well as the potential risks associated with childbirth.

Antithyroid drug (ATD) use during pregnancy carries the risk of birth defects (Level III evidence). A stable euthyroid state is indicated by two sets of normal thyroid function tests, taken at least one month apart, without any changes in therapy between tests (Level III evidence). Preconception counseling should cover treatment options for hyperthyroidism in women desiring pregnancy, including the choice between ATD treatment and definitive therapies like radioactive iodine therapy or thyroidectomy (Level III evidence).

Each treatment option has its pros and cons, which should be carefully weighed (see Table 7-1). For women preferring ATD treatment, the increased risk of birth defects associated with both propylthiouracil (PTU) and carbimazole (CMZ) should be discussed. Women well-controlled on CMZ who are planning to conceive may consider switching to PTU before pregnancy (Level III evidence). Women with thyrotoxicosis requiring high doses of ATD to maintain a euthyroid state should consider definitive treatment before pregnancy (Level III evidence). Definitive therapies like radioactive iodine or surgery have the benefit of allowing pregnancy without the teratogenic risks associated with ATD use. Conception should be delayed for at least six months after radioactive iodine therapy and only after a stable euthyroid state is achieved.

Table 7-1: Therapeutic Options for Graves' Disease Patients Planning Pregnancy (Adapted from Level III evidence)

Therapy	Advantages	Disadvantages
Antithyroid Drugs	Effective in achieving euthyroid state within 1–2 months. Often induces gradual remission of	Associated with birth defects during pregnancy. Potential adverse drug reactions. Relapse likely in 50%-70%

	autoimmunity (decreasing antibody titers). Easily adjusted or discontinued. Affordable.	of cases after discontinuation
Radioactive Iodine (RAI)	Rare chance of hyperthyroidism relapse	Rising antibody titers after treatment could worsen ophthalmopathy or pose fetal risks. Pregnancy must be deferred for at least 6 months post-RAI. A stable euthyroid state may not be reached within the first year.

		Lifelong levothyroxine therapy required.
Thyroidectomy	Definitive treatment for hyperthyroidism. Stable euthyroid state easily achieved with levothyroxine replacement.	Lifelong levothyroxine supplementation required. Surgical risks include hypoparathyroidism and recurrent laryngeal nerve injury. Gradual remission of autoimmunity after surgery.

After achieving a euthyroid state, TSH-receptor antibody (TRAb) levels may remain elevated for several months following radioactive iodine therapy. Due to this, surgery might be the preferred option for definitive treatment in patients with high TRAb levels (Level III evidence).

Recommendations:
- Women with hyperthyroidism should be informed about the importance of achieving a stable euthyroid state before attempting pregnancy. A discussion on the risks and benefits of treatment options—radioactive iodine therapy, thyroidectomy, and antithyroid drug (ATD) therapy—is essential.
- Women who require high doses of ATD to maintain a euthyroid state should consider definitive treatment before becoming pregnant.
- Women who are well-controlled on carbimazole and desire pregnancy should consider switching to propylthiouracil (PTU) before attempting conception.

Management of Graves' Disease During Pregnancy
The primary treatment for hyperthyroidism during pregnancy is the use of antithyroid drugs

(ATDs). However, the potential for teratogenic effects is a significant concern. Carbimazole is associated with aplasia cutis and carbimazole embryopathy, which includes dysmorphic facial features. Recent large studies from Japan and Denmark have revealed that carbimazole-related birth defects are more prevalent than previously thought, occurring in 1 out of 30 children exposed to the drug during gestational weeks 6–10. The identified risks include various abnormalities, such as abdominal wall defects, aplasia cutis, and atresias of the digestive, urinary, respiratory (choanal atresia), and circulatory systems (ventricular septum defects).

The Danish study also found that PTU, once considered non-teratogenic, carries a similar risk for birth defects, though the defects associated with PTU tend to be less severe. These include facial and neck malformations (preauricular sinus and cysts) and urinary tract malformations, primarily in male children. Many PTU-associated defects only become evident when the child undergoes surgery later in life, meaning studies that focus solely on birth defects at the time of birth may miss these associations.

The most critical period for teratogenicity from ATDs is gestational weeks 6–10, corresponding with organ formation. Therefore, it is essential to carefully consider treatment strategies during this time. Women undergoing ATD therapy should be encouraged to test for pregnancy regularly and contact their healthcare provider immediately if pregnancy is confirmed, so an appropriate plan can be made.

Although many patients achieve remission with ATD therapy, about half of those treated experience a relapse of hyperthyroidism after 1–2 years of medication withdrawal. Only a small percentage of patients who become TRAb-negative achieve long-term remission without further therapy.

Patients who test negative for TRAb during therapy may experience relapse within the first few months after discontinuation (Level III evidence). Therefore, stopping antithyroid drugs (ATDs) may be considered if Graves' disease is deemed in remission based on recent thyroid function tests, TRAb levels, a low dose of ATD, and overall clinical condition. After cessation of ATD, thyroid function should be closely monitored throughout the first trimester. However, ATD withdrawal is not advised for pregnant women at high risk of relapse, including those who recently started ATD therapy (within the past 6 months), still have suppressed TSH, elevated serum T3, high TRAb levels, significant goiter, active ophthalmopathy, or other signs of active disease (Level III evidence).

If ATD therapy is necessary in early pregnancy for managing overt hyperthyroidism, propylthiouracil (PTU) is preferred. Although PTU carries a risk of liver failure, this risk is lower compared to the potential for birth defects. Patients on carbimazole (CMZ) should switch to PTU early in pregnancy, using a dose ratio of

1:10 (e.g., 200 mg of PTU daily to replace 20 mg of CMZ). Due to PTU's shorter half-life, it should be administered two to three times daily (Level III evidence).

Recommendations:
- Women on ATD therapy should perform a pregnancy test as soon as a missed period is noted. If the test is positive, they should contact their healthcare provider immediately.
- During early pregnancy, consider discontinuing ATD if the patient is euthyroid on a low dose of CMZ (≤10 mg daily) or PTU (≤100 mg daily) due to potential teratogenic effects. Factors to consider before discontinuation include disease history, goiter size, duration of treatment, recent thyroid function tests, TRAb levels, and other clinical factors.
- If ATD is discontinued, thyroid function should be tested monthly, and clinical examinations should be conducted to ensure the patient remains euthyroid.

- For pregnant women who need to continue ATD, PTU is recommended throughout the first trimester.
- There is no clear recommendation regarding whether to continue PTU or switch to CMZ after the first trimester.

Monitoring Patients with Graves' Disease an STD During Pregnancy

All ATDs cross the placenta and can affect fetal thyroid function. Over-treatment of the fetus can result in fetal hypothyroidism and goiter. To minimize these risks, ATD dosage should be adjusted to maintain maternal free thyroxine (fT4) levels at or just above the pregnancy-specific upper limit of normal. The smallest effective dose of ATD should be used to manage the condition (Level III evidence).

To prevent fetal over-treatment, antithyroid drugs (ATDs) may be discontinued in the last trimester as the incidence of Graves' disease (GD) diminishes due to decreased thyroid autoimmunity (Level II-2 evidence).

In the absence of trimester-specific free thyroxine (fT4) reference ranges, the non-pregnant reference range should be used. Monitoring of fT4 levels should occur every 4–6 weeks after the initiation of therapy and upon achieving target values (Level III evidence).

Recommendations:
- Use the lowest effective dose of ATD during pregnancy, aiming to maintain fT4 levels at or just above the reference range.

The Role of Thyrotropin Receptor Antibody (TRAb) Assays in Pregnancy

Thyrotoxicosis etiology is best diagnosed by TRAb testing, where a positive result strongly suggests Graves' disease (GD).

In pregnancy, as in the non-pregnant state, elevated TRAb levels are indicative of GD (Level II evidence). GD affects 0.4%–1% of women prior to pregnancy and 0.2%–0.4%

during pregnancy, making it the most prevalent cause of hyperthyroidism in women of reproductive age (Level III evidence). TRAb levels typically decrease throughout pregnancy due to the immunosuppressive effects, often becoming undetectable by the end of the third trimester.

Table 7-2: Indications and Timing for TRAb Assays in Pregnancy

Indication for TRAb	Timing	TRAb Level at Risk for Fetal Hyperthyroidism
Previous history of Graves' illness treated by surgery or radioiodine ablation	Early in pregnancy; repeat at weeks 18–22	>3 times upper limit of normal

Patient on ATDs for treatment of Graves' hyperthyroidism when pregnancy is confirmed	Early in pregnancy	increased TRAb between weeks 18 and 22 or the mother's use of ATD throughout the third trimester Elevated TRAb at weeks 18–22 or the
Patient requires treatment with ATDs for Graves' disease through mid-pregnancy	Repeat at weeks 18–22	Elevated TRAb at weeks 18–22

| | Repeat at weeks 30–34 | |

TRAb Testing Recommendations:

In pregnant women with a history of Graves' disease (GD) or those currently managing GD, TRAb levels should be monitored. If TRAb levels are low or undetectable during early pregnancy, no further testing is necessary. However, if TRAb levels are elevated or if the patient is undergoing antithyroid drug (ATD) therapy, TRAb should be re-evaluated between weeks 18 and 22. If TRAb levels are 3–4 times above the upper limit of normal, another measurement should be taken during weeks 30–34. Maternal TRAb concentrations exceeding three times the upper limit of normal in the third trimester are associated with an increased risk of neonatal hyperthyroidism.

Recommendations:

- For patients with a history of GD treated with ablation (radioiodine or surgery), perform an initial TRAb test during early pregnancy.
- If TRAb levels are low or undetectable in early pregnancy, no further TRAb testing is necessary.
- If TRAb levels are elevated or if the patient is on ATDs, measure TRAb again between weeks 18 and 22.
- If elevated TRAb levels are found between weeks 18–22 or if the mother is on ATDs during the third trimester, conduct a further TRAb measurement in weeks 30–34 to determine the need for neonatal and postnatal monitoring.

Foetal Monitoring:

Uncontrolled hyperthyroidism and elevated TRAb levels can impact fetal well-being. Fetal hyperthyroidism should be diagnosed based on maternal history, serum TRAb levels, and fetal ultrasonography. Early signs of fetal thyroid dysfunction visible on ultrasound include fetal goiter. Additional signs of potential fetal hyperthyroidism detectable by ultrasonography include fetal tachycardia (heart rate >170 bpm), intrauterine growth restriction, accelerated bone maturation, signs of congestive heart failure, and fetal hydrops.

Recommendation:
- Foetal surveillance is advised for women with uncontrolled hyperthyroidism during the second half of pregnancy and elevated TRAb levels at any point during pregnancy (greater than three times the upper limit of normal). This monitoring should include ultrasound assessments of heart rate, growth, amniotic fluid volume, and the presence of fetal goiter.

Management of Thyrotoxicosis in Breastfeeding Patients

Antithyroid drugs (ATDs) are the primary treatment for thyrotoxicosis during the postpartum period. Both propylthiouracil (PTU) and methimazole (MMI) can be present in breast milk in minimal quantities. Research indicates that these drugs do not adversely affect the thyroid function, physical, or mental development of infants breastfed by mothers undergoing treatment for thyrotoxicosis. The largest studies have found no significant differences in the IQ or physical development of infants breastfed by mothers on ATDs compared to those who are not. Therefore, breastfeeding should be encouraged and is considered safe for mothers on ATD therapy.

Recommendation:
- When ATD is necessary, both carbimazole (CMZ) and PTU are suitable for breastfeeding mothers. The lowest effective dose should be used, as these medications transfer only a small amount into breast milk.

Chapter Eight
Postpartum Thyroiditis (PPT)

Definition and Natural History

Postpartum thyroiditis (PPT) refers to thyroid dysfunction occurring within the first year postpartum in women who were euthyroid before pregnancy. This condition often begins with transient thyrotoxicosis, followed by transient hypothyroidism, with a return to euthyroid status by the end of the postpartum year. The incidence of PPT in the general population is approximately 5.4%. Among those affected, about 22% present with the classical form, 30% with isolated thyrotoxicosis, and 48% with isolated hypothyroidism.

The thyrotoxic phase typically occurs between 2 and 6 months postpartum and resolves spontaneously. The hypothyroid phase can last from 3 to 12 months postpartum, with about 20%–40% of cases leading to permanent hypothyroidism over the subsequent 3–12 years. Studies have shown that 50% of women with PPT remain hypothyroid by the end of the first postpartum year.

Aetiology

PPT is an autoimmune disorder characterized by the presence of thyroid antibodies (TPOAb and TgAb), lymphocyte abnormalities, complement activation, elevated IgG1 levels, increased Natural Killer (NK) cell activity, and specific Human Leukocyte Antigen (HLA) haplotypes. Women with positive thyroid antibodies in the first trimester have a high risk of developing PPT, ranging from 33% to 50%. Higher antibody titres correlate with an increased risk of PPT. Histological analysis of fine-needle aspirates from PPT cases reveals lymphocytic thyroiditis.

Postpartum thyroiditis (PPT) shares similarities with silent thyroiditis in its pathophysiology. The incidence of PPT is 3- to 4-fold higher in women with type 1 diabetes mellitus and is also linked with other autoimmune conditions, including systemic lupus erythematosus (SLE) and chronic viral hepatitis. Additionally, antipituitary antibodies have been detected in 25% of women with a prior history of PPT.

Differentiation from Graves' Disease (GD) and Investigations

TSH receptor antibodies, which are positive in nearly all cases of GD, are typically negative in PPT, though mixed forms can occur. An elevated T4:T3 ratio is indicative of PPT. Physical signs associated with GD, such as goiter with a bruit or ophthalmopathy, are diagnostic when present. Radioiodine uptake studies reveal elevated or normal uptake in GD, while it is reduced during the thyrotoxic phase of PPT.

Management

During the thyrotoxic phase of PPT, symptomatic relief can be achieved with beta-blockers, such as propranolol or metoprolol, which are safe for lactating women. Treatment is generally required for a few weeks. Antithyroid drugs are not advised for managing the thyrotoxic phase of PPT.

In the hypothyroid phase, levothyroxine (LT4) should be initiated if the patient is symptomatic, lactating, or planning another pregnancy. Asymptomatic women or those with mild symptoms should have their thyroid function tests (TFT) monitored every 4 to 8 weeks until normal levels are restored. The duration for which LT4 should be continued is not well established; however, maintaining a euthyroid state is crucial for women who are pregnant or planning to conceive. LT4 dosage can be tapered starting at 12 months postpartum, with regular monitoring of TSH levels every 6 to 8 weeks to determine if the hypothyroid phase is transient or permanent.

Recommendations:

- Symptomatic women in the thyrotoxic phase of PPT should receive beta-blocker therapy. Antithyroid drugs are not recommended.
- Women in the hypothyroid phase of PPT should be treated with LT4 if symptomatic. Those not treated should have their TFT monitored every 4 to 8 weeks until euthyroid status is achieved.
- Women who are planning another pregnancy or are breastfeeding should continue LT4 treatment during the hypothyroid phase of PPT.
- LT4 dosage should be tapered after 12 months postpartum, with TFT monitored every 6 to 8 weeks.

Monitoring

After the thyrotoxic phase of postpartum thyroiditis (PPT) resolves, serum TSH levels should be checked approximately 4 to 8 weeks later or if new symptoms arise, to assess for the hypothyroid phase. Between 10% and 50% of women who initially recover from the hypothyroid phase of PPT may eventually develop permanent hypothyroidism. Factors that increase the risk of persistent hypothyroidism include multiparity, ultrasound-detected thyroid hypoechogenicity, severity of initial hypothyroidism, higher TPO antibody levels, older maternal age, and a history of pregnancy loss. Women with a previous history of PPT should have annual TSH tests to monitor for permanent hypothyroidism. For those with a prior history of PPT, additional autoimmune conditions, or positive TPO antibodies, screening at 3 months postpartum with TSH and free T4 is recommended. If results are euthyroid and TPO antibodies are negative, no further screening is needed. However, if TPO antibodies are positive but euthyroid, further TSH testing should be performed at 6 and 9 months postpartum.

Recommendations:
- Women with a history of autoimmune disorders (e.g., type 1 diabetes, SLE) should be screened for postpartum thyroiditis.

- Women with a history of postpartum thyroiditis in previous pregnancies or with positive thyroid antibody titres should be screened for PPT.
- Women with a prior history of PPT and negative TPO antibodies should have their thyroid function tested at 3 months postpartum. If normal, no additional screening is required. If TPO antibodies are positive but euthyroid, TSH should be checked at 6 and 9 months postpartum.
- Women with resolved PPT and a high risk for permanent hypothyroidism should have annual thyroid function tests to monitor for permanent hypothyroidism.
- TFT should be monitored 4 to 8 weeks after the resolution of the thyrotoxic phase to screen for the hypothyroid phase.

Postpartum Thyroiditis and Postpartum Depression

Current research does not establish a clear link between postpartum thyroiditis (PPT) and postpartum depression. Studies have yielded mixed results, with some indicating an association between thyroid antibodies and depression regardless of thyroid function, while others found no link between microsomal antibodies and postpartum depression. Given that hypothyroidism can be a treatable cause of depression, all patients with postpartum depression should be screened for thyroid dysfunction.

Recommendations for Postpartum Depression Screening
- Women with postpartum depression should be evaluated for hypothyroidism through thyroid function tests.

Acquired Hypothyroidism and Hyperthyroidism in Children and Adolescents

Prevalence of Hashimoto's Thyroiditis
Hypothyroidism is the most prevalent thyroid dysfunction among children and adolescents. The overall prevalence of hypothyroidism in individuals under 22 years old is 0.135%, with a

rate of 0.113% in those aged 11–18 years. Autoimmune thyroiditis is the most common cause of acquired hypothyroidism. Data from the National Health and Nutrition Examination Survey (NHANES III) conducted between 1988 and 1994 revealed that 6.3% of adolescents aged 12–19 had positive antithyroglobulin antibodies, while 4.8% tested positive for antithyroid peroxidase antibodies. The highest incidence of antithyroid antibodies was observed in Hispanic-American adolescents, with lower rates in black non-Hispanic adolescents, and intermediate rates in non-Hispanic white adolescents.

Clinical Features of Hashimoto's Thyroiditis
In children, the primary manifestation of hypothyroidism is a decline in height velocity, leading to short stature. This symptom often develops insidiously and may be present for several years before other symptoms emerge. Common symptoms include impaired school performance, sluggishness, lethargy, cold intolerance, constipation, dry skin, brittle hair,

facial puffiness, and muscle pain. Physical examination frequently reveals a diffusely enlarged thyroid gland (goiter) in 39.5% of cases. Other physical findings may include short stature, apparent overweight, puffy facial appearance with a dull expression, bradycardia, pseudohypertrophy of muscles, and delayed deep tendon reflexes. Pubertal development may be delayed in most cases, although some children may experience precocious puberty, characterized by breast development and vaginal bleeding in girls and macroorchidism in boys.

Recommendation:
- The clinical presentation of hypothyroidism in children and adolescents parallels that in adults. However, it is crucial to assess growth and pubertal development in children, as growth retardation and abnormal puberty are common features.

Natural History of Hashimoto's Thyroiditis in Children and Adolescents

Hashimoto's thyroiditis is observed more frequently in females than males, with a ratio of 2.8:1, and is more common among white children compared to black children. Among all affected children, euthyroid goiter is more prevalent than hypothyroidism. Typically, hyperthyroidism associated with Hashimoto's thyroiditis (Hashitoxicosis) resolves within an average of eight months. In cases where Hashimoto's thyroiditis is accompanied by euthyroidism, 64.8% of patients remain euthyroid after five years. Predictive factors for the development of hypothyroidism include the presence of goiter, elevated levels of TPO and ATG antibodies, and a progressive increase in TSH levels.

A rare outcome of Hashimoto's thyroiditis is the development of Graves' disease in approximately 7% of children and adolescents. This change is attributed to a shift in the TSH receptor antibody activity from predominantly blocking the receptor in the hypothyroid phase to stimulating it in Graves' disease.

In cases of Hashimoto's thyroiditis with subclinical hypothyroidism, 89.6% of patients exhibited thyroid dysfunction after a five-year follow-up. Increased risks of thyroid dysfunction are associated with Turner syndrome (100% in those with Turner syndrome versus 63.6% without) and Down syndrome (97.6% in those with Down syndrome versus 63.6% without). Conversely, idiopathic subclinical hypothyroidism is often benign, with 61.9% of cases returning to a euthyroid state by the end of a five-year follow-up.

Recommendation:
- Assess for goiter, measure antithyroid antibodies, and evaluate TSH patterns as these factors predict the future development of hypothyroidism.

Diagnosis and Investigation of Hashimoto's Thyroiditis in Children and Adolescents

Hashimoto's thyroiditis can be diagnosed based on a compatible clinical history and the measurement of antithyroid antibodies. High serum TPO antibodies are found in approximately 85%–90% of affected children and adolescents, while 30%–50% have positive ATG antibody levels. In a study, 9.2% of children with autoimmune thyroiditis had positive TSH receptor-blocking antibodies.

Thyroid ultrasonography and radionuclide scanning are infrequently used in children. In a study of 105 children with antibody-positive Hashimoto's thyroiditis, only one-third exhibited typical ultrasound findings at diagnosis.

Diagnosis and Investigation of Hashimoto's Thyroiditis in Children and Adolescents

When a patient presents with a markedly asymmetric goiter, a prominent nodule, or a smaller nodule that enlarges over time, a fine needle aspiration biopsy is recommended. Bone age assessment can be useful in evaluating skeletal maturity, as hypothyroidism in childhood and adolescence often results in a height age that is less than the chronological age.

Recommendations:
- Diagnose Hashimoto's thyroiditis in children and adolescents based on clinical history and confirm with antithyroid antibody measurements.
- Reserve ultrasound and isotope scans for cases where asymmetrical goiter, thyroid nodules, or malignancy are suspected.

Thyroid Function Patterns in Hashimoto's Thyroiditis in Children and Adolescents

A retrospective multicenter study involving 608 subjects revealed the following:
- 69% were pubertal, 58% were asymptomatic, 9% had chromosomal disorders (e.g., Turner syndrome, Down syndrome), and 17.6% had other autoimmune conditions.
- Of these subjects, 52.1% were euthyroid, while 47.9% had thyroid dysfunction.

- Among those with thyroid dysfunction, 41.4% had overt or subclinical hypothyroidism, and 6.5% had overt or subclinical hyperthyroidism.
- Significant factors increasing the likelihood of thyroid dysfunction included age under 10 years, prepubertal status, and chromosomal disorders.

Treatment of Hypothyroidism Due to Hashimoto's Thyroiditis in Children and Adolescents

Levothyroxine (L-T4) is the preferred treatment for children with hypothyroidism. The primary goals are to normalize growth, development, and pubertal progression. Since children metabolize L-T4 more rapidly than adults, higher daily doses are required based on weight:

- Ages 1–3 years: 4–6 mcg/kg body weight
- Ages 3–10 years: 3–5 mcg/kg body weight
- Ages 10–16 years: 2–4 mcg/kg body weight

Alternatively, the dose may be calculated based on body surface area, approximately 100 mcg/m²/day. The target TSH range is in the lower half of the reference range, ideally 0.5–2.0 mIU/L, and the target for free T4 is in the upper half of the reference range. Once growth and pubertal development are complete, thyroid hormone treatment may be discontinued, with thyroid function re-evaluated a month later. Treatment with levothyroxine typically results in reduced thyroid volume in patients with goiter.

Recommendations for Levothyroxine Treatment

- Levothyroxine is the recommended medication for managing Hashimoto's thyroiditis.
- Dosage: Determine levothyroxine dosage based on either body weight or body surface area.
- TSH Target Range: Maintain TSH levels in the lower half of the reference range.
- Free T4 Target Range: Aim for free T4 levels in the upper half of the reference range.
- Effectiveness: Levothyroxine is effective in reducing thyroid gland size or goiter.

Treatment of Non-Goitrous Euthyroid Hashimoto's Thyroiditis

Administering levothyroxine at a dose of 1.44±0.5 mcg/kg body weight in non-goitrous euthyroid Hashimoto's thyroiditis generally results in reduced thyroid volume compared to untreated controls. However, another study found no significant change in thyroid volume after three years of treatment.

Recommendations:
- Monitor thyroid volume, antithyroid antibodies, and thyroid function patterns in non-goitrous euthyroid Hashimoto's thyroiditis.
- The use of levothyroxine in non-goitrous euthyroid Hashimoto's thyroiditis remains debated.

Treatment of Euthyroid Hashimoto's Thyroiditis with Goiter

Treatment of euthyroid Hashimoto's thyroiditis with goiter with levothyroxine has been shown to reduce thyroid volume. A trial using a dose of 1.6±0.8 mcg/kg, adjusted to keep TSH within the normal range (0.4–4.0 mIU/L), resulted in decreased thyroid volume.

Recommendation:
- Levothyroxine is effective for treating euthyroid Hashimoto's thyroiditis with goiter.

Risk of Hypothyroidism in Turner Syndrome (TS)

Turner syndrome (TS) is associated with a higher risk of autoimmune conditions, particularly affecting the thyroid gland. Hashimoto's thyroiditis (HT) is the most frequently observed autoimmune disorder in girls with TS. In a study involving 41 girls with TS, 26.8% exhibited thyroid autoimmunity. Another long-term study reported that 42% of girls with TS had elevated thyroid autoantibodies, with 65% of those testing positive for autoantibodies developing hypothyroidism. In contrast, only 24% of the entire TS population developed hypothyroidism, and hyperthyroidism was found in just 2.5% of the group. Thyroid dysfunction was first detected from the age of eight years. In Japanese women with TS, over half had thyroid autoantibodies, with 57% of these having thyroid conditions: three with Graves' disease and 20 with Hashimoto's thyroiditis.

The natural progression of thyroid function in TS girls with Hashimoto's thyroiditis often shows a deterioration of thyroid status, affecting both those initially euthyroid and those with subclinical hypothyroidism. This association with TS can adversely impact the long-term prognosis of thyroid function.

Screening for Hypothyroidism in Turner Syndrome

The International Turner Syndrome Consensus Group recommends initial screening for hypothyroidism at diagnosis, followed by annual measurements of free T4 (fT4) and TSH throughout a person's life. Similarly, the TS Study Group advocates for annual thyroid function monitoring starting from as early as four years of age.

An observational study suggests that thyroid function should be assessed annually in girls with TS from age eight onward, with more frequent evaluations for those with positive thyroid autoantibodies. Other research highlights the importance of regular thyroid function monitoring due to the risk of developing hypothyroidism.

It is also noted that some women with TS may exhibit goiter or biochemical hypothyroidism even without detectable thyroid antibodies. Therefore, regular screening for thyroid function is advised, regardless of antibody status.

Recommendations:

- Screen for hypothyroidism at diagnosis and annually throughout life in individuals with Turner syndrome, starting from early childhood.
- Monitor thyroid function annually from age eight and more frequently if thyroid autoantibodies are present.
- Continue regular thyroid function assessments even in the absence of detectable thyroid autoantibodies.

Risk of Hypothyroidism in Down Syndrome (DS)

Children with Down syndrome (DS), or trisomy 21, have an increased risk of primary thyroid dysfunction, which rises with age. In Scotland, the prevalence of hypothyroidism among these children and adolescents is at least 5.7%. Studies show that the likelihood of hypothyroidism increases from 7% at diagnosis to 24% by age ten.

Subclinical hypothyroidism (SCHypo), characterized by serum TSH levels between 5 and 10 mIU/L with normal free or total T4, is also common in individuals with DS. Its prevalence ranges from 19.6% to 60% in children with trisomy 21. However, in most cases, thyroid function tends to normalize over time. In a study of 53 children with DS aged six months to five years, over 70% of those with SCHypo saw normalization of thyroid function, especially those without goiter or autoimmunity.

Screening for Hypothyroidism in Down Syndrome

Regular monitoring of thyroid function in individuals with trisomy 21 is recommended. Due to the increased risk of acquired thyroid disease, verification of newborn thyroid function screening results is crucial. Guidelines suggest repeating thyroid function tests at six and twelve months of age and annually thereafter. Monitoring should be thorough to detect thyroid dysfunction early.

Recommendations:

- Conduct regular thyroid function tests in individuals with trisomy 21.
- Repeat thyroid function tests at six and twelve months of age, and annually thereafter.

Treatment of Hypothyroidism in Down Syndrome

Treatment decisions should be made after a thorough discussion with the parents about the risks and benefits. Currently, there is insufficient evidence to recommend routine treatment for most children with hypothyroidism associated with DS.

Management of Subclinical Hypothyroidism (SCHypo) in Children

Subclinical hypothyroidism (SCHypo) is characterized by a serum TSH level below 10 mIU/L with normal total or free T4 levels. Decisions regarding the management of children with abnormal TSH or T4 levels should be made in consultation with a pediatric endocrinologist.

Recommendation:

- There is insufficient evidence to advocate for treatment in most children with SCHypo, where serum TSH is less than 10 mIU/L and TT4/fT4 levels are normal.

Risk of Hypothyroidism in Klinefelter Syndrome (KS)

Klinefelter syndrome (KS) has been associated with an increased incidence of autoimmune conditions, including hypothyroidism. Research involving adult men with KS indicates significantly higher rates of autoimmune diseases, such as autoimmune hypothyroidism, compared to the general population. Specifically, the rate ratio for autoimmune hypothyroidism in KS is 2.7. Despite this, there are no studies evaluating autoimmune diseases in children with KS.

Screening for Hypothyroidism in Klinefelter Syndrome

An expert panel from the Italian Society of Andrology and Sexual Medicine has recommended screening for primary hypothyroidism in adolescents and adults with KS. However, there is currently no established recommendation for screening in pediatric cases.

A review suggests that thyroid function should be assessed every 1–2 years starting from age ten, or earlier and more frequently if symptoms arise, due to the increased prevalence of autoimmune diseases in individuals with KS.

Recommendations:

- Given the elevated risk of autoimmune diseases in KS, thyroid function should be evaluated if symptoms suggestive of thyroid dysfunction are present.

- Thyroid function screening should be conducted at diagnosis and subsequently every 1–2 years starting from age ten.

Risk of Hypothyroidism in Prader-Willi Syndrome (PWS)

Hypothalamic dysfunction in Prader-Willi Syndrome (PWS) may elevate the risk of central hypothyroidism. Studies show a range of hypothyroidism prevalence in PWS, from 4.8% to as high as 20%–30%. A study of thyroid function in PWS patients up to two years of age revealed that 72.2% had serum TT4 or free T4 levels below the 2.5th percentile of the reference range. This indicates potential transient or persistent TRH-TSH axis dysfunction in young PWS patients. Early detection of such dysfunction is crucial due to its impact on neurological development.

Another study of 75 PWS children showed that during growth hormone (GH) treatment, free T4 levels decreased significantly to low-normal levels, while TSH levels remained stable. T3 levels were normal or elevated, suggesting an increased conversion of T4 to T3 in these children.

Screening for Hypothyroidism in Prader-Willi Syndrome

An international expert meeting in October 2006 recommended screening for thyroid function in PWS patients, including TSH, free T4, and free T3 measurements, particularly before and during GH treatment. A review also recommended screening within the first three months of life and annually, especially if the child is receiving GH therapy.

Recommendations:

- Hypothyroidism screening should be performed at diagnosis.
- PWS patients require monitoring of TSH, free T4, and free T3 levels before and during GH

treatment, due to the potential for central or peripheral hypothyroidism.

Treatment and Monitoring of Hypothyroidism in Prader-Willi Syndrome

Levothyroxine should be administered at standard replacement doses based on age and weight if hypothyroidism is diagnosed. Regular monitoring of thyroid function is essential to ensure proper management.

Diagnosis of Graves' Disease in Children and Adolescents

Graves' disease (GD) in children and adolescents may present with subtle symptoms that can persist for months or years before a diagnosis is made. Common manifestations include poor concentration, declining academic performance, irritability, fatigue, palpitations, heat intolerance, fine tremor, and goiter. In younger, prepubertal children, symptoms might include poor weight gain and frequent bowel movements, and these children are often diagnosed at a later stage. Hyperthyroidism can also impact growth, puberty, and bone density in the pediatric population. An increased rate of height growth with advanced bone age correlates with the duration of hyperthyroidism. Although bone mass may initially be reduced, it typically normalizes within two years of achieving a euthyroid state.

The thyroid gland's size may vary, but it is typically symmetrically enlarged, firm, smooth, and non-tender. Ophthalmic abnormalities are generally less severe in children compared to adults, and conditions such as thyrotoxic crisis and pretibial myxedema are rare in this age group.

The diagnosis of hyperthyroidism is confirmed with a suppressed serum TSH and elevated levels of free T4 or T3, or both. It is crucial to interpret free T4 levels according to age-specific reference ranges, as variations exist between different assay manufacturers. Some prepubertal children might exhibit isolated T3 toxicosis, with elevated serum T3 but normal free T4 levels. When a child presents with a symmetrically enlarged thyroid, recent onset of orbitopathy, and moderate-to-severe hyperthyroidism, the diagnosis of GD is likely, and further investigation into the etiology may not be necessary. If the diagnosis remains uncertain, additional diagnostic tests may include measuring TSH-receptor antibodies (TRAb), assessing radioactive iodine uptake (RAIU), or evaluating thyroid blood flow via ultrasonography. TRAb testing is particularly useful as it is a sensitive and specific biomarker for GD and reflects disease severity and activity.

Higher levels of serum TRAb are positively correlated with free T4 levels, especially in children aged 5 years or younger. TRAb measurement can aid in distinguishing GD from the toxic phase of chronic lymphocytic thyroiditis or subacute thyroiditis. However, TRAb can be negative in mild or early presentations of GD, and this may also result from assay insensitivity. Other thyroid antibodies, such as antithyroglobulin and antithyroid peroxidase, may be present but are not specific for GD.

Thyroid ultrasonography in GD typically reveals a diffusely enlarged and often homogeneous thyroid gland. Ultrasound is recommended for any patient with suspected GD to assess the thyroid gland.

Management of Graves' Disease in Children and Adolescents

Diagnosis and Evaluation

Diagnosis of Graves' disease (GD) is typically based on clinical suspicion and confirmed by elevated free T4 and/or T3 levels with suppressed TSH. It is crucial to interpret free T4 levels based on age-specific reference ranges and account for variations between different assays. In patients presenting with a symmetrically enlarged thyroid, recent onset of ophthalmopathy, and moderate-to-severe hyperthyroidism, GD is likely, and additional evaluation of the etiology may not be necessary. However, if the etiology of hyperthyroidism is unclear, measuring TSH receptor antibodies is recommended as they are specific to GD.

Thyroid ultrasound should be performed if there is thyroid gland asymmetry or a palpable nodule. If a significant nodule is identified, fine-needle aspiration biopsy and a thyroid scan should be considered. Although rare, differentiated thyroid cancer (DTC) can occur alongside GD or an autonomous nodule, and adolescents with GD have been reported to present with DTC. Given the uncertainty about the increased risk of malignancy in nodules found in autoimmune thyroid disease, a thorough evaluation is advised. Radioisotope imaging is not necessary for diagnosing GD but may be useful if the etiology is unclear, if TSH receptor antibodies are negative, or if the clinical presentation suggests a thyroid adenoma or multinodular goiter.

Recommendations

- Diagnosis of GD is confirmed by clinical evaluation along with elevated free T4 and/or T3 levels and suppressed TSH.
- Free T4 levels should be interpreted according to age-specific reference ranges and variations in assay methodologies.
- In cases with a symmetrically enlarged thyroid, recent onset of ophthalmopathy, and moderate-to-severe hyperthyroidism, GD is likely, and further etiology investigation may be unnecessary.
- If the etiology is uncertain, measuring TSH receptor antibodies is recommended as they are specific for GD.
- Ultrasound is recommended for patients with thyroid gland asymmetry or palpable nodules.

Treatment Options

Three primary treatment options for GD include antithyroid drugs (ATD), radioiodine therapy (RAI), and thyroidectomy.

1. Antithyroid Drugs (ATD):
    - First-line treatment involves ATDs, specifically carbimazole or its active metabolite methimazole (MMI). Propylthiouracil should generally be avoided in children due to the risk of idiosyncratic liver failure.
    - The typical dosage for methimazole/carbimazole ranges from 0.2 to 0.5 mg/kg daily, with a usual starting dose of 0.5 to 1 mg/kg/day and a maximum of 30 mg/day. High initial doses (>30 mg for adolescents or adults) are rarely used due to dose-related side effects that often occur within the first three months.
    - Methimazole/carbimazole can be administered once daily, which enhances compliance, though divided dosing has not been shown to be more effective. For rapid biochemical control in severe thyrotoxicosis, an

initial split dose of MMI/carbimazole may be used.

2. Radioiodine Therapy (RAI)
3. Thyroidectomy

Management and Monitoring of Graves' Disease in Children and Adolescents

Medication Dosage and Administration

Methimazole or carbimazole, typically administered at 0.2–0.5 mg/kg daily (with a range of 0.1 mg/kg to 1.0 mg/kg daily and a maximum initial dose of 30 mg/day), is the first-line treatment for Graves' disease (GD). While a single daily dose is common, a divided dose (e.g., 15 mg twice daily) may be more effective due to the medication's duration of action being less than 24 hours. Beta-blockers, such as atenolol, propranolol, or metoprolol, are recommended for managing significant symptoms like tachycardia, muscle weakness, tremor, or neuropsychological changes. In patients with asthma or reactive airway disease, cardio-selective beta-blockers (atenolol or metoprolol) should be used with caution.

Treatment Regimens and Alternatives

Meta-analyses indicate that the block-and-replace regimen has a higher incidence of adverse events compared to dose titration. This is likely due to higher doses of methimazole/carbimazole and associated dose-related complications, thus this approach should not be routinely employed. Propylthiouracil (PTU) is generally reserved for short-term use in cases where patients have adverse reactions to methimazole or are not candidates for radioiodine therapy or surgery. PTU poses a higher risk of idiosyncratic liver failure, occurring in approximately 1 in 2000–4000 children.

Recommendations

- Initial Treatment: The first-line treatment for GD is antithyroid drugs (ATD), specifically methimazole or carbimazole.
- Dosage: Typical dosing is 0.2–0.5 mg/kg daily, with a range from 0.1 mg/kg to 1.0 mg/kg daily and a maximal initial dose of 30 mg/day.
- Dose Adjustment: After 2–4 weeks, when thyroid hormone levels normalize, reduce the initial dose by 30%–50%.
- TSH Levels: TSH levels may take 2–4 months to appear in the serum and should not be used for dose titration.
- Avoidance of PTU: Propylthiouracil should be avoided in children except in specific situations due to the risk of liver failure.
- Block-and-Replace Regimen: This regimen should not be routinely used.
- Beta-Blockade: Consider beta-adrenergic blockers for children with significant hyperthyroid symptoms, especially tachycardia. Use cardio-selective beta-blockers cautiously in patients with asthma or reactive airway disease.

Monitoring Antithyroid Drug Therapy

Once thyroid hormone levels have normalized (typically after 2–4 weeks), the initial dose of antithyroid drugs should be gradually reduced by 30%–50%. Hypothyroidism may occur if the dose is not adjusted as serum free T4 levels normalize. TSH levels, which can take 2–4 months to become detectable, should not be used for dose adjustment. Initially, thyroid function should be monitored every 2–6 weeks following the initiation of antithyroid drug therapy.

Monitoring and Managing Side Effects of Antithyroid Drugs

Medication Dosage and Adjustments

When adjusting carbimazole dosage, options include one tablet (5 mg), half a tablet (2.5 mg), or a quarter tablet (1.25 mg) for infants. Once the dose is stabilized, thyroid function should be monitored every 2–3 months.

Liver Function Monitoring and Side Effects

Propylthiouracil (PTU) can cause rapid and severe liver damage; routine liver function tests have not proven effective in predicting PTU-related liver injury. Methimazole (MMI) and carbimazole are more commonly associated with side effects in the initial 3–6 months of treatment, often linked to higher doses. Minor reactions, such as rash, urticaria, arthralgia, and gastrointestinal issues, occur in 5%–25% of cases. Agranulocytosis, though rare, affects approximately 0.2% to 0.5% of patients.

Side Effects Summary

- Minor Reactions: Rash, pruritus, hives, hair loss, nausea, decreased taste, joint pain, and arthralgia.
- Severe Reactions: Agranulocytosis, neutropenia, thrombocytopenia, Stevens-Johnson syndrome, cholestatic jaundice, hepatitis.

Stevens-Johnson syndrome has been reported in 3 out of 100 patients on MMI, typically at doses exceeding 30 mg/day. The incidence of severe side effects is low in patients receiving MMI at doses below 10 mg/day.

Patient Education and Monitoring

Patients should be informed of potential side effects, ideally in writing, and advised to seek medical attention if symptoms such as pruritic rash, jaundice, acholic stools, dark urine, arthralgias, abdominal pain, nausea, fatigue, fever, or pharyngitis develop. Prior to starting antithyroid drug (ATD) therapy, a baseline complete blood count (CBC) and liver profile, including bilirubin, transaminases, and alkaline phosphatase, should be obtained. Although routine WBC count monitoring is not generally recommended due to the rarity and sudden onset of agranulocytosis, WBC counts should be measured during febrile illnesses or at the onset of pharyngitis.

Management of Propylthiouracil (PTU) and Antithyroid Drug Therapy in Children

Use of Propylthiouracil (PTU)
PTU is generally not recommended for children. If used, it should be discontinued immediately if the child exhibits symptoms such as anorexia, pruritus, rash, jaundice, light-colored stool, dark urine, joint pain, right upper quadrant pain, abdominal bloating, nausea, or malaise. Liver function should be assessed in these cases, and PTU should be stopped if transaminase levels exceed 2–3 times the upper limit of normal. Following discontinuation, liver function tests, including bilirubin, alkaline phosphatase, and transaminases, should be monitored weekly. If liver function does not improve, referral to a hepatologist is advised.

Monitoring and Managing Weight and Side Effects
Children receiving antithyroid drugs (ATDs) should have their weight monitored regularly, as

excessive weight gain is common and may persist. Persistent mild cutaneous reactions to methimazole (MMI) should be managed with antihistamines or by discontinuing MMI and considering alternative treatments such as radioactive iodine (RAI) or surgery. In cases of serious adverse reactions to an ATD, switching to another ATD is not recommended. Instead, RAI or surgery should be considered due to the higher risks associated with PTU compared to these alternatives.

Special Circumstances

In situations where there is a risk of thyroid storm and an ATD is needed for a child with severe adverse reactions to MMI, PTU may be used temporarily to control hyperthyroidism. In such cases, families should be fully informed of the associated risks of PTU.

Recommendations

- Initial Monitoring: Thyroid function should be checked every 2–6 weeks initially, and subsequently every 2–3 months once the dose is stabilized.

- Dose Considerations: High doses of MMI (>30 mg/day for adolescents or adults) should be avoided initially due to the risk of dose-related side effects occurring within the first three months of treatment.

- Baseline Testing: A baseline complete blood count (CBC), including WBC count with differential, and liver function tests (LFT) should be performed before starting ATD therapy. Routine monitoring of CBC and LFT is not recommended due to the unpredictable onset of adverse effects.

- White Blood Cell Monitoring: Measure WBC counts if the child develops fever, arthralgia, mouth sores, pharyngitis, or malaise, and consider withholding ATDs if needed.

- Patient and Caregiver Education: Inform patients and caregivers about potential adverse effects of ATDs, ideally in writing.

- Management of Cutaneous Reactions: Persistent minor skin reactions to MMI should be managed with antihistamines or by discontinuing the medication and switching to RAI or surgery. For serious adverse reactions to ATDs, alternative treatments should be considered rather than switching to another ATD.

Use of Propylthiouracil (PTU) in Children

PTU is generally contraindicated in children due to its associated risks. If PTU is administered, it should be discontinued immediately if the child exhibits symptoms such as anorexia, pruritus, rash, jaundice, light-colored stool, dark urine, joint pain, right upper quadrant pain, abdominal bloating, nausea, or malaise. Liver function should be assessed promptly in these cases.

Indications for Definitive Therapy

Definitive treatment options for Graves' Disease (GD) include radioactive iodine (RAI) and thyroidectomy. These therapies are considered in cases of relapse after an adequate trial of antithyroid drugs (ATDs), non-compliance, or adverse effects from ATDs. The timing for considering definitive therapy after initiating ATD treatment is debated.

According to the American Thyroid Association's 2016 guidelines, pediatric patients with GD who do not achieve remission after 1–2 years of methimazole (MMI) or carbimazole should be evaluated for definitive treatment. MMI or carbimazole can be continued beyond this period if the patient tolerates the medication without adverse effects. Patients and their caregivers should be informed about all available therapeutic options to make a well-informed decision.

Remission rates with ATD therapy after 1–2 years are generally low, around 20%–30%, defined as remaining euthyroid for one year after discontinuation of therapy. However, a French study reported remission rates of 20%, 37%, 45%, and 49% after 4, 6, 8, and 10 years of follow-up, respectively, for children treated with ATD. Therefore, while definitive therapy is recommended after 1–2 years of ATD, continuing treatment for a longer duration may be appropriate if well-tolerated.

Retrospective studies indicate that the likelihood of remission after two years of ATD treatment is lower in the presence of certain factors, such as a large thyroid gland (more than 2.5 times the normal size for age), young age (<12 years), prepubertal status, non-Caucasian ethnicity, high serum TSH receptor antibody (TRAb) levels during therapy, and significantly elevated free T4 levels (>50 pmol/L) at diagnosis.

Table 8-1:Predictors of Poor Remission

Predictor	Description
Large thyroid gland	Greater than 2.5 times the normal size for age
Young age	Less than 12 years

Prepubertal status	Prepubertal
Non-Caucasian ethnicity	Non-Caucasian
High serum TRAb levels	Elevated TRAb levels during therapy
Elevated free T4 levels	Free T4 levels >50 pmol/L at diagnosis

Persistence of Graves' Disease (GD) in Children

The persistence of GD in children is often associated with elevated levels of TSH receptor antibodies (TRAb). While low TRAb levels might not guarantee remission, monitoring TRAb levels during antithyroid drug (ATD) treatment can be useful in adults for predicting remission or relapse. This method's effectiveness in children has not yet been validated.

Recommendations

- Definitive treatments for GD include radioactive iodine (RAI) and thyroidectomy.
- Indications for considering definitive therapy in children are relapse after an appropriate period on ATDs, issues with compliance, or adverse effects from ATDs.
- Children who do not achieve remission after two years on methimazole (MMI) or carbimazole should be evaluated for RAI or thyroidectomy.
- MMI or carbimazole may be continued beyond two years if the hyperthyroid condition is managed effectively without side effects.
- Patients on long-term ATD therapy should be reassessed every 6–12 months and during the transition to adulthood.

Clinical Considerations for RAI Therapy

The American Thyroid Association (ATA) 2016 guidelines advise against using RAI in children under five years old due to the increased risk of thyroid gland sensitivity to ionizing radiation. RAI may be considered for children aged five to ten if the administered dose is less than 10 mCi (473 MBq).

When RAI is used, it should be given in a dose sufficient to make the patient hypothyroid to minimize the risk of residual thyroid tissue, which could potentially develop into thyroid neoplasms.

Children with GD who have total T4 levels greater than 20 ng/dL (260 nmol/L) or free T4 levels exceeding 5 ng/dL (60 pmol/L) should be pretreated with MMI or carbimazole and a beta-blocker until T4 levels normalize before RAI administration. Although the exact incidence of worsening hyperthyroidism after pretreatment is unclear, there are rare cases of severe hyperthyroidism leading to thyroid storm post-RAI.

For children on MMI or carbimazole scheduled for RAI, these medications should be discontinued 2–3 days before the RAI treatment. Beta-blockers should be administered until T4 levels normalize after RAI therapy. Thyroid hormone levels in children typically start to decrease within the first week after RAI and may take 2–4 months to normalize.

Use of Antithyroid Drugs (ATDs) After Radioactive Iodine (RAI) Therapy

While some physicians may resume ATD therapy following RAI, this practice is rarely necessary in children.

RAI Administration and Dosage

The dosage of RAI should be based on thyroid gland size and uptake rather than age. Reducing the RAI dose due to age can lead to undertreatment and the need for additional RAI sessions, increasing overall radiation exposure. For patients with large goiters, the RAI dose is typically higher. It is crucial to accurately estimate gland size to avoid insufficient RAI administration. In cases where the goiter exceeds 80 grams, surgery may be a more suitable option than RAI.

Dosing Strategies

Some medical centers administer a fixed RAI dose for all children, while others calculate the dose based on gland size. Ultrasonography is recommended to assess thyroid size, particularly for large glands. There is insufficient data comparing the outcomes of fixed versus calculated RAI doses in children. Calculated dosing may allow for lower administered RAI while ensuring effectiveness.

Post-Therapy Monitoring

RAI is excreted through saliva, urine, sweat, tears, and stool, with significant radioactivity retained in the thyroid for several days. Patients and families should be advised on local radiation safety guidelines. After RAI therapy, T3, T4, and/or free T4 levels should be monitored monthly. TSH levels may remain suppressed for several months post-treatment and thus may not be useful for monitoring. Hypothyroidism typically develops 2–3 months after successful RAI therapy and should be managed with levothyroxine.

Side Effects and Risks

Side effects from RAI therapy in children are generally infrequent, with lifelong hypothyroidism being a primary outcome. Less than 10% of children may experience thyroid tenderness in the first week post-treatment, which can be managed with acetaminophen or NSAIDs for 24–48 hours.

Long-Term Considerations

There is a theoretical risk of thyroid cancer from residual thyroid tissue in young children following RAI, based on observations from historical radiation exposure studies such as those after Hiroshima and Chernobyl. This risk appears age-dependent, with the highest risk for children under 5–6 years old. However, these observations may not directly apply to RAI therapy risk assessments. Additionally, factors such as iodine deficiency and exposure to different radionuclides might have contributed to cancer risks observed after the Chernobyl incident. In contrast, thyroid cancer rates did not increase among children exposed to RAI in an iodine-sufficient region, such as Hanford.

Use of Antithyroid Drugs (ATDs) After Radioactive Iodine (RAI) Therapy

While resuming ATD therapy following RAI may be considered by some physicians, it is generally unnecessary in children.

RAI Administration and Dosage

RAI dosage should be determined based on the size and uptake of the thyroid gland, rather than the patient's age. Adjusting the dose to account for age can lead to inadequate treatment and the potential need for additional RAI, thus increasing overall radiation exposure. For patients with large goiters, higher RAI doses are often required. Accurate assessment of thyroid size is essential to prevent underdosing. For goiters larger than 80 grams, surgical intervention may be preferred over RAI.

Dosing Strategies

Medical centers may use either a fixed RAI dose for all children or adjust the dose based on gland size. Ultrasonography is recommended for evaluating large thyroid glands. There is limited data comparing fixed versus calculated RAI dosing outcomes in children. Calculated dosing may allow for more precise treatment with potentially lower radiation doses while ensuring effectiveness.

Post-Therapy Monitoring

RAI is excreted through various bodily fluids and retains significant radioactivity in the thyroid for several days. It is important to follow local radiation safety guidelines. Following RAI therapy, T3, T4, and/or free T4 levels should be monitored monthly. TSH levels may remain suppressed for months after treatment and are not reliable for monitoring. Hypothyroidism usually develops 2–3 months after successful RAI therapy and should be managed with levothyroxine.

Side Effects and Risks

RAI therapy in children usually has few side effects, with lifelong hypothyroidism being the most common outcome. Less than 10% of children may experience thyroid tenderness during the first week after treatment, which can be managed with acetaminophen or NSAIDs for 1–2 days.

Long-Term Considerations

Theoretical risks of thyroid cancer from residual thyroid tissue following RAI are based on studies of historical radiation exposure, such as those from Hiroshima and Chernobyl. The risk appears highest for children under 5–6 years of age. However, these historical data may not directly correlate with RAI therapy risks. Other factors, such as iodine deficiency and exposure to different radionuclides, may have influenced cancer rates after the Chernobyl incident. Studies have shown no increased thyroid cancer rates among children exposed to RAI in iodine-sufficient regions, such as Hanford.

Long-Term Risk of Non-Thyroid Malignancies After RAI Therapy

Long-term studies of children treated with radioactive iodine (RAI) for Graves' disease (GD) have not demonstrated an increased risk of non-thyroid malignancies. Identifying such a risk would require a study with over 10,000 children treated before the age of 10, which is likely more than the number of such treated children. Theoretical projections suggest a potential low risk of malignancies from low-level, whole-body radiation exposure in very young children treated with RAI.

Recommendations:
- RAI therapy should generally be avoided in children younger than 5 years.
- RAI may be considered for children aged 5 to 10 years if the dose required for treatment is less than 10 mCi (<370 MBq).
- When RAI therapy is used for GD, the dose should be sufficient to render the patient hypothyroid in a single administration.
- RAI may be indicated in young children under certain conditions, such as adverse reactions to ATDs, lack of surgical expertise, or if the child is not a suitable candidate for surgery.
- For children with GD who have total T4 levels greater than 260 nmol/L or free T4 levels above 60 pmol/L, pretreatment with MMI and beta-adrenergic blockers is recommended until these levels normalize before starting RAI therapy.

Clinical Considerations for Thyroidectomy

Thyroidectomy is the preferred definitive treatment for GD in very young children (under 5 years) when performed by an experienced thyroid surgeon. It is also the treatment of choice for individuals with large thyroid glands (greater than 80 grams), where RAI may be less effective. A total or near-total thyroidectomy is recommended. Preoperative treatment typically includes MMI for 1–2 months. Iodides, such as potassium iodide (50 mg iodide/drop), may be administered 1–2 drops three times daily for ten days before surgery, mixed in juice or milk.

Children have a higher rate of surgical complications compared to adults, including an increased risk of transient hypoparathyroidism. Postoperative calcium levels should be monitored, and treatment with calcitriol and calcium supplements may be necessary. Intravenous calcium infusions for postoperative hypocalcemia occur more frequently in children than adults. The complication rate is also higher with less experienced surgeons. High-volume centers with experienced thyroid surgeons report lower complication rates for thyroidectomy in children.

Recommendations for Thyroidectomy in Young Children:

- Preferred Treatment: Thyroidectomy is the recommended treatment for Graves' disease in very young children (under 5 years) when definitive therapy is necessary.
- Large Thyroid Glands: Thyroidectomy should also be considered for patients with large thyroid glands (greater than 80 grams) where radioactive iodine (RAI) might be less effective.
- Surgical Approach: If surgery is chosen, a total or near-total thyroidectomy is advised.
- Referral: It is recommended to refer children requiring thyroidectomy to a specialized center with extensive expcricncc in pediatric thyroid surgery.
- Preoperative Preparation: Children undergoing thyroidectomy should be made euthyroid using

MMI or carbimazole. Potassium iodide drops should be administered in the preoperative period.

- Postoperative Care: Younger children are at higher risk for hypoparathyroidism after surgery. Calcium levels should be monitored, and treatment with calcitriol and calcium supplements may be necessary.

- Multidisciplinary Management: Care should involve a multidisciplinary team, including experienced thyroid surgeons, pediatric endocrinologists, and anesthesiologists.

Thyroid Disorders in the Elderly

Features of Overt Hyperthyroidism in the Elderly:

- Atypical Presentation: Elderly patients may not exhibit classical hyperthyroid symptoms such as tremor, weight loss, palpitations, diarrhea, and heat intolerance. Instead, they may present with symptoms of "apathetic thyrotoxicosis," including depression, lethargy, and weight loss.

- Thyrotoxic Encephalopathy: Some elderly patients may display agitation and confusion, indicative of "thyrotoxic encephalopathy."
- Nonspecific Symptoms: Fatigue, weakness, agitation, confusion, dementia, and myopathy are often misinterpreted as normal aging changes. These nonspecific symptoms are more commonly observed in smokers and those with elevated free T4 levels.

Treatment of Overt Hyperthyroidism in the Elderly:

- Medication Efficacy: A randomized controlled trial comparing MMI alone versus MMI combined with a beta-adrenergic blocker showed that patients taking the beta-blocker had lower heart rates, reduced shortness of breath, less fatigue, and improved physical functioning as measured by the SF-36 health questionnaire.
- Diagnosis and Management: Once hyperthyroidism is confirmed and attributed to Graves' disease, treatment should be tailored to the patient's needs and medical condition.

Initial Treatment Options for Hyperthyroidism

Patients with hyperthyroidism can choose from three effective and relatively safe initial treatment options: radioactive iodine (RAI) therapy, antithyroid drugs (ATDs), or thyroidectomy. Research indicates that the long-term quality of life (QoL) is similar among patients randomly assigned to any of these treatment modalities. Currently, there is no scientific evidence supporting the use of alternative therapies for hyperthyroidism.

Recommendations

- Beta-Adrenergic Blockade: Recommended for all patients with symptomatic thyrotoxicosis, particularly the elderly and those with resting heart rates exceeding 90 beats per minute or coexisting cardiovascular conditions.
- Treatment Modalities: For overt Graves' disease, any of the following treatments may be considered: RAI therapy, ATDs, or surgery.

- Surgical Indications: Surgery is advised in the following situations:
  - Presence of symptomatic compression or large goiters (>80 grams).
  - Low uptake of RAI.
  - Documented or suspected thyroid malignancy (e.g., suspicious or indeterminate cytology).
  - Large thyroid nodules, particularly those larger than 4 cm or showing hypofunction on imaging.
  - Coexisting hyperparathyroidism requiring surgical intervention.
  - Extremely high TRAb levels.
  - Moderate to severe active Graves' Ophthalmopathy (GO).
- Surgical Contraindications: Surgery is not recommended for patients with significant comorbidities such as severe cardiopulmonary disease, end-stage cancer, or other debilitating conditions, or when access to an experienced thyroid surgeon is limited.
- RAI Treatment Considerations: Given that RAI can transiently worsen hyperthyroidism, beta-adrenergic blockade should be considered

even for asymptomatic patients at higher risk for complications due to this worsening.

- Long-Term MMI Use: For elderly patients, those with limited life expectancy, or those not suitable for surgery or ablative therapy, long-term MMI treatment for toxic multinodular goiter (TMNG) or toxic adenoma (TA) might be a viable option.

Risks of Subclinical Hyperthyroidism in the Elderly

The impact of subclinical hyperthyroidism on clinical outcomes remains uncertain and debated. Risks associated with untreated subclinical hyperthyroidism include the potential progression to overt hyperthyroidism and an increase in overall mortality.

Association of Subclinical Hyperthyroidism with Health Risks

Subclinical hyperthyroidism has been linked to various health risks, including cardiovascular disease, arrhythmias, osteoporosis, and fractures. It is associated with cognitive impairment, frailty, and an increased risk of mild cognitive impairment and dementia in elderly individuals. Even a slight excess of thyroid hormone can lead to reduced physical function in older men. Additionally, elderly individuals at high cardiovascular risk with low or very high TSH levels and normal free T4 levels are at increased risk for developing heart failure.

In older adults with endogenous subclinical hyperthyroidism and TSH levels between 0.1 mIU/L and 0.4 mIU/L, the progression to clinical hyperthyroidism is rare (approximately 1% annually), and spontaneous normalization of TSH levels may occur. Subclinical hyperthyroidism often persists for many years. Men with subclinical hyperthyroidism are at a higher risk for hip fractures, with lower serum TSH levels linked to an increased risk of such fractures. Lower TSH levels within the euthyroid range are associated with reduced bone mineral density (BMD) and weaker femoral structure in elderly women, with low TSH levels independently correlating with decreased BMD at the femoral neck in women without overt thyroid dysfunction. Subclinical hyperthyroidism is also an independent risk factor for all-cause mortality in older adults.

However, studies of well-functioning elderly individuals have found no evidence that subclinical thyroid dysfunction affects functional capacity or contributes to cognitive decline. There is no consistent evidence that subclinical thyroid disorders affect cognitive impairment, physical function, depression, or mortality in the elderly. For example, elderly individuals with subclinical hyperthyroidism did not show significantly worse survival compared to their euthyroid counterparts. Additionally, subclinical thyroid disorders did not impact the risk of hip fractures, BMD, or left ventricular mass progression during a five-year follow-up in older individuals.

Management of Subclinical Hyperthyroidism in the Elderly

Subclinical hyperthyroidism may progress to overt hyperthyroidism and is associated with increased cardiovascular and skeletal risks. The impact of subclinical hyperthyroidism may vary based on TSH suppression levels, underlying causes, patient age, and duration of TSH suppression. Recent meta-analyses indicate that subclinical hyperthyroidism is linked to higher risks of coronary heart disease mortality, atrial fibrillation, heart failure, and fractures.

Excess Mortality and Treatment Recommendations for Subclinical Hyperthyroidism in the Elderly

Patients with serum TSH levels below 0.1 mIU/L are at an increased risk of excess mortality, including serious cardiovascular events and fractures. Although randomized prospective trials are lacking, evidence suggests that treating patients over 65 with TSH levels below 0.1 mIU/L may help mitigate these risks and prevent progression to overt hyperthyroidism. In patients over 65 with TSH levels between 0.1 and 0.39 mIU/L, treatment should be considered if they exhibit symptoms of hyperthyroidism or have underlying conditions such as heart disease, diabetes, renal failure, previous stroke or transient ischemic attack, left atrial dilation, or increased risk factors for cardiovascular events.

Recommendations
- Treatment for subclinical hyperthyroidism (SCHyper) is advised for all individuals aged 65 and older with persistently low TSH levels (<0.1 mIU/L).
- For individuals aged 65 and older with TSH levels below the normal range but ≥0.1 mIU/L, consider treatment if they have cardiac disease, osteoporosis, or symptoms of hyperthyroidism.

Management of Subclinical Hyperthyroidism in the Elderly

The approach to treating subclinical hyperthyroidism is similar to that for overt hyperthyroidism. Treatment should be guided by the underlying cause of thyroid dysfunction and follow the principles applied to overt hyperthyroidism. Radioactive iodine (RAI) is suitable for most patients, particularly older individuals where toxic multinodular goiter (TMNG) is a common cause of subclinical hyperthyroidism. However, there is limited data on whether elderly patients with subclinical hyperthyroidism would benefit from pretreatment with antithyroid drugs (ATDs) before RAI therapy. The potential risks of ATD therapy may outweigh any minor benefits due to the low risk of exacerbation.

ATD therapy is a reasonable alternative to RAI, especially for younger patients with Graves' disease (GD) and subclinical hyperthyroidism, as remission rates are higher in those with milder disease.

Recommendations

- In patients older than 65 with GD and TSH levels between 0.1 and 0.4 mIU/L, antithyroid drugs should be the first-line treatment due to observed remission rates in 40%–50% of patients with overt hyperthyroidism 12–18 months post-treatment.

- Consider RAI therapy if ATDs are not tolerated, if there is a relapse, or if the patient has cardiac disease.

- For patients older than 65 with GD and TSH levels <0.1 mIU/L, especially those with cardiac disease, either ATDs or RAIL should be used to manage high-risk patients and prevent adverse cardiac events.

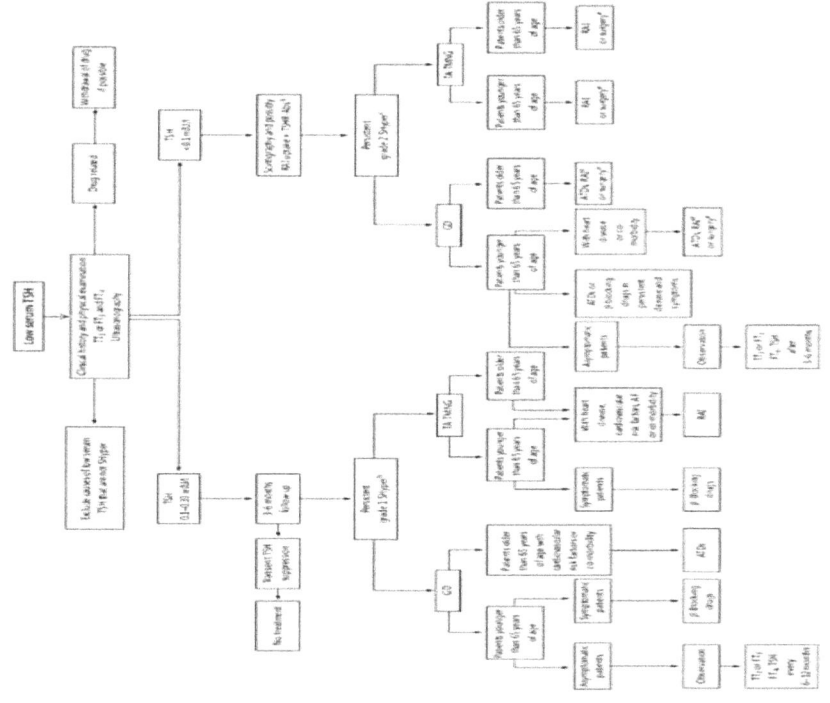

Management of Subclinical Hyperthyroidism and Hypothyroidism in the Elderly

Subclinical Hyperthyroidism

For patients over 65 years with subclinical hyperthyroidism (SCHyper) caused by multinodular goiter (MNG) or toxic adenoma (TA), radioactive iodine therapy (RAI) or surgery are the preferred treatment options due to the likelihood of persistent SCHyper.

- If RAI is not feasible—such as in elderly patients in nursing homes who may be incontinent or those with severe comorbidities, a growing goiter, or pressure symptoms—long-term low-dose antithyroid drugs (ATDs) may be considered.
- Surgery is advised for patients with SCHyper who have a large goiter, symptoms of compression, coexisting hyperparathyroidism, or suspected thyroid malignancy. Total thyroidectomy is recommended when there are no complicating conditions.

Overt Hypothyroidism

Elderly patients are more susceptible to the adverse effects of excessive thyroid hormone, including atrial fibrillation and osteoporotic fractures. Therefore, careful dose titration of levothyroxine (LT4) is crucial to avoid iatrogenic thyrotoxicosis.

- Initiate levothyroxine treatment with a small dose, such as 25 or 50 µg daily. Increase the dose by 25 µg/day every 14–21 days until the full replacement dose is achieved.
- For older patients (aged >70–75 years), a higher target for serum TSH, around 1–5 mIU/L, is acceptable due to the higher normal TSH ranges in this age group.

Subclinical Hypothyroidism

Subclinical hypothyroidism (SCHypo) carries risks including progression to overt hypothyroidism, mood disturbances, heart failure, dyslipidemia, cardiovascular disease (CVD), and increased mortality. SCHypo is associated with a heightened risk of incident heart failure and persists for up to four years in over half of older individuals, with higher rates of reversion to euthyroidism in those with lower TSH levels and negative thyroid peroxidase antibodies (TPO Ab). Both SCHypo and subclinical hyperthyroidism are linked to increased mortality in the elderly, with a TSH threshold (>6.35 mIU/L) indicating a higher mortality risk. However, the impact of SCHypo on cardiovascular events is less clear in moderately older individuals (<70–75 years) and may diminish in those over 80–85 years.

Evaluation and Management of Subclinical Hypothyroidism in the Elderly

Several studies have shown that subclinical hypothyroidism (SCHypo) does not always lead to adverse outcomes. There is no increased risk of coronary heart disease (CHD), heart failure (HF), or cardiovascular death in older adults with persistent SCHypo. Elevated TSH levels, particularly those above 10 mIU/L, are linked to increased CHD events; however, this association is less pronounced in the elderly, especially those over 85 years of age, who have lower mortality rates. SCHypo does not seem to be associated with an elevated risk of metabolic or neuropsychological issues in older individuals. Moreover, those with moderate SCHypo exhibit similar mobility and decline rates as euthyroid individuals. Studies also find no significant link between SCHypo or subclinical hyperthyroidism and hip fracture risk or bone mineral density (BMD) in older adults. Similarly, there is no conclusive evidence that subclinical thyroid dysfunction impacts mortality in older men. Research indicates that higher TSH and lower free T4 (fT4) concentrations within the euthyroid range may be associated with a lower risk of adverse events, suggesting that lower thyroid hormone levels might be well-tolerated in the elderly. Additionally, SCHypo does not appear to cause significant mood or cognitive impairments in most older patients, and those aged 85 with SCHypo and subclinical hyperthyroidism do not experience significantly worse survival compared to euthyroid peers.

Management Recommendations for Subclinical Hypothyroidism in the Elderly

There is no evidence supporting the benefit of T4 replacement therapy for improving cognitive function in elderly individuals with SCHypo. Levothyroxine treatment has shown no apparent advantages in Hypothyroid Symptom Scores for older adults with SCHypo.

Management Algorithm for SCHypo

- Age ≤70 Years:
  - Serum TSH <10 mIU/L: Monitor and repeat thyroid function tests (TFTs) in 6 months.
  - Serum TSH ≥10 mIU/L: Assess for hypothyroid symptoms. If symptoms are present, start a 3-month trial of levothyroxine (LT4) and then evaluate the response. If no symptoms are evident, monitor and repeat TFTs in 6 months.

- Age >70 Years:
  - Serum TSH <10 mIU/L: Monitor and repeat TFTs in 6 months.
  - Serum TSH ≥10 mIU/L: Consider LT4 treatment if there are clear symptoms of hypothyroidism or if the patient has high vascular risk.

Cardiovascular Impact and Management of Subclinical Hypothyroidism in the Elderly

The negative effects of subclinical hypothyroidism (SCHypo) on cardiovascular events and mortality are well-documented in younger adults but are less pronounced in individuals aged 70–75 years. In those older than 80–85 years, these effects may diminish. Further randomized controlled trials (RCTs) evaluating levothyroxine treatment for SCHypo, particularly focusing on hard cardiovascular endpoints across different age groups, are needed.

Recommendations:

- For patients over 70 years old with serum TSH levels ≥10 mIU/L, consider initiating levothyroxine therapy if there are clear symptoms of hypothyroidism or high vascular risk.

- For patients over 70 years old with serum TSH levels ≤10 mIU/L, observe and repeat thyroid function tests (TFTs) in 6 months.
- For patients 70 years old or younger with serum TSH levels ≥10 mIU/L, consider levothyroxine treatment.
- For patients 70 years old or younger with serum TSH levels ≤10 mIU/L and symptoms of hypothyroidism, consider a three-month trial of levothyroxine, then assess the response.
- For patients 70 years old or younger with serum TSH levels ≤10 mIU/L and no symptoms of hypothyroidism, observe and repeat TFTs in 6 months.

Management of Subclinical Hypothyroidism in the Elderly:

The approach to treating subclinical hypothyroidism in the elderly should align with the principles used for overt hypothyroidism. Treatment should be individualized, gradual, and closely monitored. For individuals over 70 years old, aiming for a higher serum TSH target (approximately 1–5 mIU/L) is acceptable.

Drug-Induced Thyroid Disorders

Amiodarone-Induced Thyroid Disease

Thyroid Abnormalities Induced by Amiodarone:

Amiodarone, a benzofuran derivative with a structural formula similar to that of thyroxine (T4), contains about 37% iodine by weight. Each day, approximately 10% of the drug's iodine is deiodinated, releasing 7–21 mg of iodide daily due to a maintenance dose ranging from 200 to 600 mg. This results in a significant increase in urinary iodine excretion, providing 50- to 100-fold excess iodine daily.

In euthyroid patients taking amiodarone, serum thyroxine (T4) and free T4 levels typically increase by 20%–40% within the first month of therapy, while serum triiodothyronine (T3) levels may decrease by up to 30% within the initial weeks. Serum reverse T3 concentrations usually rise by 20% shortly after starting treatment. Serum thyroid-stimulating hormone (TSH) levels may also slightly increase and can exceed the upper normal limit after three to six months of therapy.

Thyroid Function During Amiodarone Therapy

In most patients who were euthyroid at baseline, thyroid function reaches a steady state during amiodarone treatment. Typically, serum TSH levels normalize, while total T4, free T4, and reverse T3 levels may remain slightly elevated or within the upper normal range, and serum T3 levels often stay at the low end of the normal range. Approximately 15%–20% of patients on amiodarone develop thyroid dysfunction, manifesting as either thyrotoxicosis (amiodarone-induced thyrotoxicosis, AIT) or hypothyroidism (amiodarone-induced hypothyroidism, AIH). Thyroid dysfunction can arise at any point during treatment. AIH often occurs early, particularly in those with preexisting chronic autoimmune thyroiditis, while AIT can emerge at any time during treatment or even months after discontinuation due to the slow release of the drug and its metabolites. Monitoring thyroid function periodically, including after discontinuing amiodarone, is recommended.

Recommendation:

- Conduct thyroid function tests (TFTs) before initiating amiodarone, 3–4 months after starting the medication, and subsequently at 3–6 month intervals. Continue monitoring for up to 1 year after stopping amiodarone.

Mechanisms and Diagnosis of Amiodarone-Induced Thyrotoxicosis (AIT)

Amiodarone-induced thyrotoxicosis (AIT) can occur in patients with preexisting thyroid conditions (type 1) or in those with normal thyroid glands (type 2). AIT is characterized by suppressed TSH levels with elevated free T4 and/or free T3 levels.

- Type 1 AIT: This form is iodine-induced hyperthyroidism resulting from excessive thyroid hormone production in response to increased iodine, often seen in individuals with nodular goiter or latent Graves' disease.
- Type 2 AIT: This is a destructive thyroiditis affecting otherwise normal thyroid tissue and is more common in iodine-sufficient areas.
- Mixed/Indefinite Type: This type displays characteristics of both AIT 1 and AIT 2.

Accurate diagnosis of AIT subtypes is crucial for determining the appropriate treatment. Thyroid ultrasonography can help identify the presence of a diffuse or nodular goiter, while color Doppler ultrasound is more reliable, showing absent hypervascularity in AIT 2 and increased vascularity in AIT 1. Nuclear imaging with thyroid 131I uptake (RAIU) can further differentiate between types, with AIT 2 typically showing very low RAIU (<3%) and AIT 1 displaying low-normal to increased uptake. Alternative tracers such as 99mTcO4 and 99mTcO4 2-methoxy-isobutyl-isonitrile (MIBI) may also be utilized.

Management of Amiodarone-Induced Thyrotoxicosis (AIT)

Type 1 AIT: This form of hyperthyroidism, caused by an excess of iodine, is effectively managed with antithyroid medications. Due to the reduced sensitivity of an iodine-saturated thyroid to , higher doses are necessary (40–60 mg/day of methimazole or equivalent doses of carbimazole or propylthiouracil). Treatment durations may range from 4 weeks to 3–6 months to achieve euthyroidism. In regions where potassium or sodium perchlorate is available, these can be used in doses of up to 1 g daily for 4–6 weeks to expedite control of hyperthyroidism.

Type 2 AIT: This form is best treated with corticosteroids such as prednisolone.

Improvement is often observed within a few weeks, sometimes as early as one week. A study comparing treatments for Type 2 AIT showed that prednisolone alone restored euthyroidism in all patients, whereas 30% of those receiving only sodium perchlorate required additional prednisolone. Prior data indicated that prednisolone alone achieved euthyroidism in 76% of patients, compared to 15% with methimazole alone. The recommended dose of prednisolone is typically 40 mg daily for 2–4 weeks, followed by a gradual taper over 2–3 months based on clinical response.

Mixed or Indefinite AIT: In cases where the exact type of AIT cannot be determined, two strategies can be considered. The first involves initiating treatment with (and possibly sodium perchlorate) as for Type 1 AIT. If there is no biochemical improvement within 4–6 weeks, glucocorticoids can be added, assuming a destructive component is present alongside an underlying thyroid disorder. Alternatively, a combined approach using both and glucocorticoids from the start can be employed. The optimal treatment for mixed or indefinite AIT remains uncertain, and further randomized clinical trials are needed. Lithium has been studied as a treatment option, but its efficacy is limited and unconfirmed. Radioiodine therapy is typically not effective due to low thyroidal iodine uptake. Patients unresponsive to medical treatment may require thyroidectomy, which has shown to improve cardiac function in severe cases of left ventricular dysfunction without causing mortality.

The decision to continue or discontinue amiodarone in patients with AIT should be individualized. Continuing amiodarone may increase the risk of recurrent thyrotoxicosis, delay stabilization of euthyroidism, and prolonged exposure to excess thyroid hormones. This decision must be made based on the specific circumstances of each patient.

Management of Amiodarone-Induced Thyrotoxicosis (AIT)

Continued Use in Critical Cases: Amiodarone may be continued in critically ill patients with life-threatening cardiac conditions that respond to the medication and in cases of Type 2 AIT, as this form often resolves on its own.

Recommendations:
- Type 1 AIT: Treat with high-dose carbimazole, 40 mg daily or its equivalent.
- Type 2 AIT: Manage with corticosteroids, specifically prednisolone at 40 mg daily for 2–4 weeks, followed by a gradual taper over 2–3 months.
- Mixed or Indefinite AIT: If monotherapy is ineffective or the distinction between Type 1 and Type 2 AIT is unclear, use a combination of carbimazole and corticosteroids.
- Unresponsive Cases: For patients who do not respond to aggressive medical treatment, consider thyroidectomy.
- Amiodarone Use: The decision to continue or stop amiodarone should be individualized and discussed with the cardiologist.

Management of Amiodarone-Induced Hypothyroidism (AIH)

AIH presents similarly to hypothyroidism from other causes, although goiter is rare. Risk factors include underlying chronic autoimmune thyroiditis and female gender. AIH may present as subclinical or overt hypothyroidism and is typically managed with levothyroxine (LT4). There is no need to discontinue amiodarone if it is essential for treating the underlying cardiac condition. However, treatment for subclinical hypothyroidism might be unnecessary in the elderly due to potential cardiovascular risks. Regular thyroid function tests every 4–6 months are recommended to monitor progression. If amiodarone is stopped, adjust LT4 dosage to avoid overtreatment, as AIH may resolve in approximately 50% of cases within 2–3 months.

Recommendation:
- Overt AIH: Initiate LT4 treatment in all cases.

Other Drugs Causing Thyroid Disorders

- Interferon-alpha (IFN-α): Used mainly for treating hepatitis C, IFN-α can cause thyroid dysfunction in 1% to 35% of patients, with the risk being higher in those with pre-existing thyroid antibodies. Studies indicate that approximately 50% of patients with positive thyroid peroxidase antibodies before treatment develop thyroid dysfunction compared to 5.4% of those without such antibodies.

Thyroid Dysfunction Associated with Interferon-alpha (IFN-α)

In patients without thyroid antibodies, thyroid dysfunction is less common. However, positive thyroid antibodies with normal thyroid function tests are frequently observed during IFN-α treatment. During therapy, patients may develop antithyroglobulin antibodies (Anti-Tg) and TSH receptor antibodies (TRAb). Clinical manifestations can include painless thyroiditis, Hashimoto's thyroiditis, or Graves' disease.

Changes in thyroid function tests typically emerge after three months of therapy but can occur at any time during treatment.

According to Hwang et al., the average time to develop thyroid dysfunction is about 18 weeks post-treatment. A recent study involving 1,233 euthyroid patients at baseline reported that 16.7% developed abnormal TSH levels: 4.6% had suppressed TSH, 5.7% had hypothyroidism, and 6.4% developed biphasic thyroiditis. The average onset times for these conditions were 17.5 weeks for thyrotoxicosis, 18.9 weeks for biphasic thyroiditis, and 22.7 weeks for hypothyroidism.

Management of thyroid dysfunction during IFN-α therapy depends on the underlying condition: Graves' disease is treated with antithyroid medications, the thyrotoxic phase of thyroiditis is managed with beta-blockers if symptomatic, and symptomatic hypothyroidism is treated with levothyroxine. Discontinuation of IFN-α is generally not required but may be considered in severe thyrotoxicosis cases, with consultation from a hepatologist recommended.

Recommendations:
- Monitor thyroid function tests before starting treatment and at least 3–4 months after initiation.
- Check for thyroid antibodies to rule out Graves' disease and Hashimoto's thyroiditis if available.
- Manage thyroid disorders induced by IFN-α and IL-2 according to their etiology (refer to management guidelines for thyroiditis, Graves' disease, and hypothyroidism).
- Discontinuation of IFN-α and IL-2 is usually not necessary.

Thyroid Dysfunction Associated with Interleukin-2 (IL-2)

Patients with metastatic cancer and leukemia undergoing IL-2 treatment may experience thyroid dysfunction, including thyroiditis, hypothyroidism, and hyperthyroidism. Hypothyroidism occurs in 20%–50% of patients receiving IL-2, and most affected individuals have positive thyroglobulin or thyroid peroxidase antibodies. There have been reports of thyroid storms following IL-2 initiation with the development of TRAb. Treatment of IL-2-induced thyroid dysfunction follows similar protocols as those for IFN-α-induced thyroid disorders.

Recommendations:
- Monitor thyroid function tests before treatment and at least every 3–4 months during therapy.
- Check thyroid antibodies to exclude Graves' disease and Hashimoto's thyroiditis if available.
- Manage thyroid disorders induced by IL-2 based on their etiology (refer to management guidelines for thyroiditis, Graves' disease, and hypothyroidism).
- Discontinuation of IL-2 is generally not necessary.

Thyroid Dysfunction Associated with Tyrosine Kinase Inhibitors (TKIs)

Tyrosine kinase inhibitors (TKIs) such as sunitinib, sorafenib, and nilotinib are used to treat various malignancies, including metastatic renal cell carcinoma, hepatoma, thyroid cancers, and gastrointestinal stromal tumors (GIST). Sunitinib is reported to induce hypothyroidism in 36%–85% of patients, while sorafenib induces it in 23.1%–67.7% of patients. The mechanisms of thyroid dysfunction associated with TKIs include direct effects on the thyroid gland and interference with thyroid hormone metabolism.

Thyroid Dysfunction Associated with Tyrosine Kinase Inhibitors (TKIs)

Tyrosine kinase inhibitors (TKIs) such as sunitinib and sorafenib are associated with thyroid dysfunction, including hypothyroidism and destructive thyroiditis. For example, in a study of 69 patients receiving sorafenib for metastatic renal cell carcinoma, 66.7% developed hypothyroidism, either initially or following destructive thyroiditis. The median time to abnormal thyroid function tests with sorafenib was 1.7 months.

In another study of 31 patients treated with sunitinib for metastatic renal cell carcinoma, 19.3% developed thyrotoxicosis, with one case progressing to thyroid storm. The onset of thyrotoxicosis occurred between 4 and 15 weeks after starting sunitinib. Thyroid antibodies did not correlate with the development of thyroiditis.

Management of TKI-induced thyroiditis includes beta-blockers, with or without NSAIDs, for mild thyrotoxicosis, and glucocorticoids for severe cases. Symptomatic hypothyroidism should be treated with levothyroxine. There are no established guidelines or randomized controlled trials (RCTs) recommending the discontinuation of TKIs for thyrotoxicosis. However, discontinuation was reported in 2 out of 5 cases of severe thyrotoxicosis in a case series.

Recommendations:

- Evaluate thyroid function at baseline and monitor every 4–12 weeks thereafter, or sooner if symptoms arise.
- Manage TKI-induced thyroiditis and hypothyroidism according to existing guidelines for thyroiditis and hypothyroidism.
- Discontinuation of TKIs is usually unnecessary.

Thyroid Dysfunction Associated with Lithium

Patients on lithium for bipolar disorder are at increased risk of thyroid dysfunction, including both hypothyroidism and, less frequently, thyrotoxicosis. Published series indicate that the incidence of thyrotoxicosis ranges from 0.6% to 3.0% of patients. The primary cause of hyperthyroidism in these cases is destructive thyroiditis, though Graves' disease and toxic nodular goiter have also been reported. Destructive thyrotoxicosis is typically managed conservatively with beta-blockers, while corticosteroids are avoided due to the risk of triggering manic episodes.

Lithium can also inhibit thyroid hormone release, leading to goiter and hypothyroidism. The annual incidence of goiter in patients on continuous lithium therapy is about 4%. The prevalence of hypothyroidism ranges from 6% to 52%, with a higher risk in older women and those with thyroid antibodies.

Management of lithium-induced hypothyroidism involves levothyroxine, while goiter is managed similarly to other cases of goiter. Discontinuation of lithium is generally not required.

Recommendations:
- Monitor thyroid function tests before initiating lithium therapy and annually thereafter, or every 6 months for older women with thyroid antibodies.

Recommendations for Managing Thyroid Dysfunction Related to Lithium:

- Monitoring: Assess thyroid function tests (TFTs) before starting lithium therapy and every 6–12 months thereafter.
- Goitre Management: Follow established guidelines for goiter management.
- Hypothyroidism Management: Treat with levothyroxine (refer to the section on hypothyroidism management).
- Hyperthyroidism Management: Address based on the underlying cause, including thyroiditis, Graves' disease, or toxic multinodular goiter.
- Discontinuation of Lithium: Discontinuation is generally not required if thyroid dysfunction occurs.

Recommendations for Managing Thyroid Dysfunction Related to Immune Checkpoint Inhibitors (ICIs):

Immune checkpoint inhibitors, including CTLA-4 inhibitors (e.g., ipilimumab), PD-1 inhibitors (e.g., nivolumab, pembrolizumab), and PD-L1 inhibitors (e.g., atezolizumab, avelumab, durvalumab), can lead to thyroid disorders among other endocrine issues. Thyroid dysfunction is a common adverse effect of ICIs.

- Monitoring: Check thyroid function tests at the beginning of ICI therapy and every 4–6 weeks during treatment.
- Hypothyroidism Management: For mild asymptomatic cases, continue monitoring TFTs closely. For moderate to severe cases, initiate levothyroxine therapy.
- Hyperthyroidism Management: For mild asymptomatic cases, monitor TFTs regularly. For moderate symptoms, use beta-blockers for relief and evaluate for Graves' disease if symptoms persist beyond 6 weeks. Severe cases or thyroid storms should be managed accordingly.
- Discontinuation of ICIs: Generally, discontinuation is not required unless thyroid dysfunction is severe.

Chapter Nine
Graves' Ophthalmopathy

Incidence of Graves' Ophthalmopathy

Graves' ophthalmopathy (GO), also known as thyroid-associated orbitopathy, thyroid-associated ophthalmopathy, or thyroid eye disease, has a prevalence of 34.7% in Malaysia. This rate is comparable to the 25%–50% prevalence reported in Caucasian populations. The condition typically presents with rapid deterioration followed by gradual improvement, although some residual symptoms may persist. Common symptoms observed locally include exophthalmos, upper eyelid retraction, and restrictive extraocular myopathy. Risk factors for GO include smoking, with smokers having an odds ratio of 2.75 for developing the condition, male gender, and unstable thyroid function, particularly hypothyroidism.

Definition of Graves' Ophthalmopathy

Graves' ophthalmopathy is diagnosed if there is eyelid retraction accompanied by thyroid dysfunction, exophthalmos, optic nerve dysfunction, or extraocular muscle involvement. In the absence of eyelid retraction, GO is defined by the presence of thyroid dysfunction along with either exophthalmos, optic nerve dysfunction, or extraocular muscle involvement.

Early Symptoms of Graves' Ophthalmopathy:

- Redness in the eyes or eyelids
- Swelling or fullness in one or both upper eyelids
- Eyelid edema
- Protruding or "staring" eyes (thyroid stare)
- Pain in or behind the eyes

Key Diagnostic Indicators for Graves' Ophthalmopathy:

- Recent onset thyroid dysfunction (within the last 18 months)
- Symptoms not alleviated by topical antibiotics
- Abnormal eyelid positioning (retraction of upper or lower lids)
- New swelling in the upper or lower eyelids
- Changes in eye appearance, such as protrusion
- Presence of additional signs such as diplopia (double vision) and lagophthalmos (inability to close the eyes completely)

Assessment of Activity and Severity

The clinical activity score (CAS) is the preferred method for assessing GO activity and severity. The CAST includes:

1. Spontaneous retrobulbar pain
2. Pain during upward and downward eye movements

Assessment of Graves' Ophthalmopathy Severity

Clinical Activity Score (CAS):

1. Redness of eyelids
2. Redness of conjunctiva
3. Swelling of the caruncle or plica
4. Swelling of eyelids
5. Swelling of conjunctiva (chemosis)

Scoring for Graves' Ophthalmopathy Activity:

- Inactive GO: CAS <3
- Active GO: CAS ≥3

Severity Assessment Approaches:

1. NOSPECS Classification:

   - No signs or symptoms: No evidence of GO.
   - Only signs, no symptoms: Includes lid aperture measurement (distance between lid margins in mm with the patient in the primary position, seated, with fixed distance).
   - Soft tissue involvement: Includes swelling or redness of the eyes.

- Proptosis: Measures exophthalmos in mm using a Hertel exophthalmometer, with consistent intercanthal distance for each patient.

- Extraocular muscle involvement: Assesses muscle ductions in degrees and subjective diplopia (intermittent, inconstant, or constant).

- Corneal involvement: Evaluates the presence of punctate keratopathy or ulcers.

- Sight loss: Assesses best corrected visual acuity, color vision, optic disc health, relative afferent pupillary defect, and visual fields if optic nerve compression is suspected.

2. EUGOGO Classification:

- Mild Graves' Ophthalmopathy: Symptoms minimally affect daily life and do not warrant immunosuppressive or surgical treatment. Features may include:
  - Minor lid retraction (<2 mm)
  - Mild soft tissue involvement
  - Exophthalmos <3 mm above normal for race and gender
  - No or intermittent diplopia

- Corneal exposure responsive to lubricants

- Moderate-to-Severe Graves' Ophthalmopathy: Significant impact on daily life, potentially justifying immunosuppressive or surgical intervention. Features may include:
- Lid retraction ≥2 mm
- Moderate-to-severe soft tissue involvement
- Exophthalmos ≥3 mm above normal for race and gender
- Inconstant or constant diplopia

Sight-Threatening Graves' Ophthalmopathy:

Patients with sight-threatening Graves' ophthalmopathy include those with dysthyroid optic neuropathy (DON) or corneal breakdown. Accurate categorization of Graves' ophthalmopathy (GO) involves determining whether it is active or inactive and its severity—mild, moderate-to-severe, or sight-threatening.

Recommendation:

- Assessment of GO should include evaluating both activity and severity using standardized criteria. GO is classified as active or inactive, and further categorized as mild, moderate, severe, or sight-threatening.

When to Refer to Specialists:

- Referral to an ophthalmologist or endocrinologist is necessary for all cases of GO except mild cases. It is also important to refer to cases where the diagnosis of GO is uncertain.
- Urgent referral is required if GO is sight-threatening, indicated by symptoms such as unexplained vision deterioration, changes in color vision, globe subluxation, corneal opacity, significant lagophthalmos, or disc swelling.

Treatment for Graves' Ophthalmopathy:

Non-Specific Treatment and Risk Factor Modification:

- General management includes avoiding cigarette smoke (both active and passive), and promptly restoring euthyroidism while avoiding hypothyroidism. Antithyroid medications and thyroidectomy do not appear to impact the natural progression of GO. Radioactive iodine treatment may slightly increase the risk of worsening GO or causing new onset GO, particularly in smokers, those with severe hyperthyroidism, or recent onset hyperthyroidism.
- Ocular surface inflammation and dry eyes are common in GO. To address these issues, the use of preservative-free artificial tears with osmoprotective properties, such as sodium hyaluronate, or eye lubricant gels/ointments is recommended.

Recommendations:
- Patients with Graves' disease should be advised to cease smoking.
- Euthyroidism should be promptly achieved in patients with GO.

- Ocular surface disease is prevalent and should be managed with appropriate topical therapy.

Mild Graves' Ophthalmopathy

For patients with mild Graves' ophthalmopathy (GO), a watchful approach is generally adequate. It is important to focus on non-specific treatment strategies and modifying risk factors as outlined previously.

Sodium selenite, at a dose of 100 mcg twice daily (equivalent to 93.6 mcg of elemental selenium per day) for 6 months, has demonstrated improvements in eye symptoms and quality of life (QoL) and can help prevent disease progression. The benefits of selenium supplementation were sustained even after discontinuation at 6 months. This finding comes from a large multicenter, randomized, double-blind, placebo-controlled trial. However, the participants in this study were from an area with marginal selenium deficiency. For long-standing, inactive mild GO, there is no evidence supporting the effectiveness of selenium.

In cases where mild GO significantly impacts QoL, despite being objectively mild, it may be categorized as moderate-to-severe GO, and treatment options such as immunosuppressive therapy or rehabilitative surgery should be considered (refer to the section on moderate-to-severe GO).

Recommendation:
- Topical treatments and controlling risk factors are fundamental. Selenium supplementation at 100 mcg twice daily for 6 months may be considered.

Moderate-to-Severe and Active Graves' Ophthalmopathy

First Line Treatment

High-dose intravenous glucocorticoids (GCs) are the recommended first-line treatment for moderate-to-severe active GO. The total cumulative dose of GCs should not exceed 8 grams, with a single dose not surpassing 0.75 grams, and consecutive-day therapy should be avoided. Intravenous GCs are generally better tolerated and more effective compared to oral GCs, with adverse event rates of 39% versus 81% ($p<0.001$) and response rates of 70%-80% versus 50%, respectively.

Contraindications for systemic GCs include recent viral hepatitis, significant hepatic dysfunction, severe cardiovascular conditions, uncontrolled hypertension, or psychiatric disorders. Caution is advised for diabetic and hypertensive patients. During treatment, proton pump inhibitors should be used to prevent peptic ulcers, and bone protection therapy should be considered for patients at risk of osteoporosis.

A recommended regimen involves a cumulative dose of 4.5 grams of intravenous methylprednisolone, starting with 0.5 grams weekly for 6 weeks, followed by 0.25 grams weekly for an additional 6 weeks. For more severe cases, a higher cumulative dose of 7.5 grams of methylprednisolone can be administered, starting with 0.75 grams weekly for 6 weeks, followed by 0.5 grams weekly for another 6 weeks.

Recommendation:
- High-dose intravenous glucocorticoids are the first-line treatment for moderate-to-severe active GO. The dosage should be carefully managed to avoid exceeding recommended limits, and potential contraindications should be assessed.

In a randomized, single-blind controlled trial, 35 patients with untreated, active, moderate-to-severe Graves' ophthalmopathy (GO) were administered intravenous methylprednisolone (0.5 g weekly for 6 weeks, followed by 0.25 g weekly for an additional 6 weeks). Another 35 patients received oral prednisolone (0.1 g/day, tapered by 0.01 g/week, with a cumulative dose of 4 g over 12 weeks). After 3 months, 77% of patients in the intravenous group showed improvement compared to 51% in the oral group (p<0.01). Side effects were reported in 17% of the intravenous group versus 51% of the oral group (p=0.005).

In another study involving 159 patients with active, moderate-to-severe GO, participants were randomized to receive cumulative doses of intravenous methylprednisolone: 2.25 g (Low Dose), 4.98 g (Medium Dose), or 7.47 g (High Dose) over 12 weekly infusions. At 12 weeks, improvement in ophthalmic symptoms was observed in 52% of the high-dose group compared to 35% of the medium-dose group (p=0.03) and 28% of the low-dose group (p=0.01). Clinical Activity Score (CAS) improvements were 83% for high-dose, 81% for medium-dose, and 58% for low-dose. Major adverse reactions were more frequent in the high-dose group. The study concluded that while high-dose intravenous methylprednisolone offers greater short-term benefits, it also comes with increased side effects. The intermediate dose regimen is generally preferred, reserving high doses for the most severe cases of GO.

Recommendations:
- Administer an intermediate dose of intravenous methylprednisolone at 0.5 g weekly for 6 weeks, followed by 0.25 g weekly for another 6 weeks (total cumulative dose of 4.5 g) for most cases of moderate-to-severe GO.
- Reserve high-dose regimens of intravenous methylprednisolone (0.75 g weekly for 6 weeks, followed by 0.5 g weekly for 6 weeks, with a cumulative dose of 7.5 g) for the most severe cases.
- Ensure the cumulative dose of intravenous methylprednisolone does not exceed 8 g.
- Assess for viral hepatitis, liver function, cardiovascular issues, blood glucose levels, and blood pressure before starting intravenous methylprednisolone.

Second-Line Treatment:
- Consider a second course of intravenous glucocorticoids if the cumulative dose of 8 g

methylprednisolone is not exceeded and the patient tolerates the treatment well.

- Orbital radiotherapy may be considered, especially for improving diplopia and eye movement range in moderate-to-severe GO cases. Orbital radiotherapy, typically administered as a cumulative dose of 20 Gy over 10 daily fractions within 2 weeks, has been shown to enhance the effects of systemic glucocorticoids.

- Combining cyclosporine with glucocorticoids has been found to be more effective than either treatment alone in active, moderate-to-severe GO, according to randomized controlled studies.

In a study, patients were treated with prednisolone at 100 mg per day, tapering the dose over 3 months, either alone or in combination with cyclosporine at 5 mg/kg per day for 12 months. The combination therapy showed significantly better ocular outcomes and a lower rate of GO recurrence compared to prednisolone alone. Another trial indicated that while prednisolone alone was more effective than cyclosporine alone, the combination therapy produced the best results. Common adverse effects associated with cyclosporine include dose-dependent liver and renal toxicity as well as gingival hyperplasia.

Rituximab: Data on rituximab's efficacy in treating GO are mixed. One small randomized controlled trial found that rituximab (2000 mg and 500 mg) significantly reduced GO activity compared to intravenous glucocorticoids (7.5 g), with 100% in the rituximab group showing inactivation versus 69% in the glucocorticoid group ($p<0.04$). Additionally, no disease reactivation occurred with rituximab compared to 31% in the glucocorticoid group ($p=0.043$). Conversely, another small randomized, double-masked, placebo-controlled study found no additional benefit from rituximab over placebo.

Recommendation:

- Decision-making regarding second-line therapy for moderate-to-severe GO should involve shared decision-making with the patient.

Sight-Threatening Active Graves' Ophthalmopathy:
Sight-threatening GO includes dysthyroid optic neuropathy (DON), severe corneal exposure, corneal breakdown, and eyeball subluxation. Recent choroidal folds causing metamorphopsia also require urgent attention.

Treatment Recommendations:
- For DON, administer very high doses of intravenous glucocorticoids (500–1000 mg of methylprednisolone) for 3 consecutive days or on alternate days during the first week. This regimen may be repeated after a week if needed. If there is a poor response to high-dose glucocorticoids, consider urgent decompression surgery.
- Predictors of poor response include disc swelling at diagnosis and persistent active disease 2 weeks after high-dose glucocorticoids.

- Aggressive treatment for severe corneal exposure is essential to prevent corneal breakdown. This may involve medical therapy or surgical intervention.

Recommendation:
- For dysthyroid optic neuropathy, initiate treatment with very high doses of intravenous glucocorticoids (500–1000 mg of methylprednisolone) for 3 consecutive days or on alternate days during the first week. This regimen should be repeated in the second week. If there is no improvement or the response is inadequate, proceed with urgent orbital decompression.

Moderate-to-Severe and Inactive Graves' Ophthalmopathy:
Confirming the inactivity of Graves' ophthalmopathy (GO) can be challenging. If there is any uncertainty, monitor the condition over time. Rehabilitative surgery should only be considered after the disease has been inactive for at least 6 months.

Rehabilitative Surgery Options:

1. Decompression Surgery:

 - A minimally invasive approach is preferred. This surgery aims to reduce intraocular pressure by enlarging the bony orbit through various methods, such as extending the medial/lateral orbital walls or removing the orbital floor. Fat excision from the inferolateral or inferomedial extraconal compartments is another option. Orbital decompression can alleviate exophthalmos, periorbital puffiness, lid retraction, and retro-orbital pain. It can also improve strabismus and address visual obscuration caused by orbital and optic nerve microvasculopathy. Potential complications include new or worsening strabismus and globe dystopia.

2. Strabismus Surgery:

 - This surgery aims to restore proper eye alignment and fusion in the primary position, prevent diplopia on downward gaze, and correct residual incompatibility.

3. Eyelid Surgery:

   - Medical therapies like alpha-blocker eye drops or postganglionic adrenergic blockers have limited effectiveness or are associated with significant side effects. Botulinum injections offer only temporary relief. Surgical options for lid retraction include sutureless mullerectomy, transconjunctival free en bloc recession of the levator palpebrae muscle and conjunctiva, and transcutaneous blepharotomy.

Cosmetic Periorbital Surgery:

   - These procedures are similar to those used for age-related facial changes.

If multiple surgical procedures are required, the recommended sequence is orbital decompression first, followed by strabismus surgery, and then eyelid surgery.

Recommendation:

- Elective rehabilitative surgery should be considered for patients with Graves' ophthalmopathy (GO) only after the disease has been inactive for a minimum of 6 months, especially when GO significantly impacts visual function or quality of life. Such patients should be referred to specialized centers with surgeons experienced in addressing the specific needs of each individual.

Radioactive Iodine Therapy and Graves' Ophthalmopathy:

- Radioactive iodine (RAI) therapy carries a minor yet definite risk of exacerbating pre-existing GO or triggering new onset GO. Concurrent use of glucocorticoids has been shown to mitigate the risk of worsening in patients with mild active eye disease. However, there is insufficient evidence to support the use of prophylactic glucocorticoids for nonsmokers without clinical evidence of GO undergoing RAI therapy.

- For patients with active, moderate-to-severe, or sight-threatening GO, antithyroid drugs and thyroidectomy are preferred over RAI therapy. In cases of significant but inactive GO, RAI therapy can be administered without prophylactic glucocorticoids.

Table 9-1: Recommendations for Radioactive Iodine (RAI) Therapy with or without Glucocorticoids

Condition	RAI without Glucocorticoids	RAI with Oral Glucocorticoids
No GO, nonsmoker	Recommended	Not recommended
No GO, smoker	Insufficient data	Insufficient data
GO present, active, mild,	Acceptable	Acceptable

without risk factors		
GO present, active, mild, with risk factors	Not recommended	Recommended
GO present, active, moderate-to-severe or sight-threatening	Not recommended	Not recommended
GO present, inactive	Recommended	Not recommended

Notes:

- Risk Factors: Include elevated TRAb levels, smoking, and active progressive GO in the last 3 months.
- The choice to use concurrent glucocorticoids should be guided by a careful evaluation of the

risk-benefit ratio for each patient. While glucocorticoids can help prevent deterioration of GO in the presence of risk factors, they may exacerbate conditions such as diabetes, hypertension, osteoporosis, psychiatric disorders, and increase infection risk.

Prednisolone Dosage for GO Prophylaxis

For patients with mild-to-moderate Graves' ophthalmopathy (GO), the recommended dosage of prednisolone for prophylaxis is 0.4–0.5 mg/kg per day, starting 1–3 days after radioactive iodine (RAI) therapy. This regimen should be maintained for one month, followed by a gradual tapering over the subsequent two months. Studies indicate that 15% of patients receiving RAI developed or experienced worsening of GO within 2–6 months, while none in the RAI and prednisolone group showed progression. A lower dose of 0.2–0.3 mg/kg per day for six weeks may be effective for patients with milder GO or those without GO prior to RAI but with significant risk factors.

Recommendations:

- For patients with active, moderate-to-severe or sight-threatening GO, surgery or antithyroid medications are preferred.

- Oral prednisolone at 0.4 -- 0.5 mg/kg per day for a total of three months is recommended for patients with mild-to-moderate GO undergoing RAI therapy.

- A lower dose of 0.2–0.3 mg/kg per day can be considered for patients with milder GO or those with risk factors.

Figure 9-2: Management Strategy for Graves' Ophthalmopathy (GO).

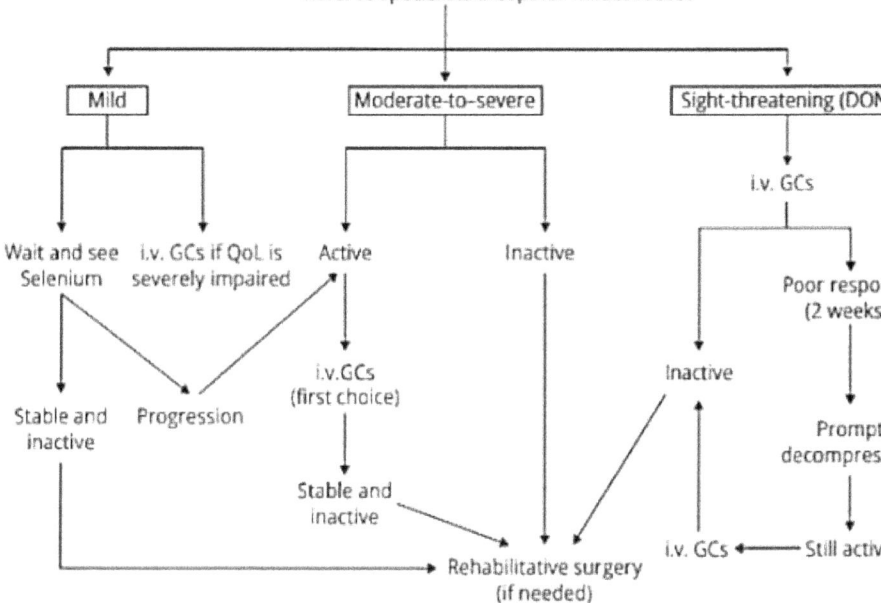

Chapter Ten
Implementation of Clinical Practice Guidelines (CPG)

Implementing Clinical Practice Guidelines (CPG) is essential for delivering high-quality healthcare based on the best available evidence tailored to local conditions and expertise. Successful adoption of CPG recommendations requires addressing various facilitating and limiting factors, as well as understanding resource implications.

Facilitating and Limiting Factors

Facilitating Factors:
- Availability of CPG in both printed and digital formats for healthcare providers.
- Regular conferences and updates on thyroid disorder management organized by professional societies such as the Malaysian Endocrine and Metabolic Society, Family Medicine Specialist

Association, and the Academy of Family Physicians Malaysia.
- Public awareness campaigns on thyroid diseases, such as those held on World Thyroid Day.

Limiting Factors:
- Variability in care levels and practices due to differences in expertise, facilities, and financial resources.
- Limited awareness among high-risk populations regarding thyroid disease.

Potential Resource Implications

Successful implementation of the CPG involves:
- Ensuring the CPG is widely distributed to healthcare providers.
- Providing ongoing training through effective seminars and workshops.
- Engaging a multidisciplinary team at all levels of healthcare.

Proposed Clinical Audit Indicators for Quality Management:

- Proportion of patients with euthyroid hyperthyroidism or hypothyroidism:

  - Formula: (Number of patients with euthyroid hyperthyroidism/hypothyroidism / Total number of patients with hyperthyroidism/hypothyroidism) × 100%

  - Target: > 80%

Key Recommendations

Dr. Yoshiki Kiyomizu have highlighted the following primary clinical recommendations for implementation:

Hyperthyroidism

- For patients suspected of hyperthyroidism, obtain serum TSH and free T4 (fT4) levels during the initial assessment. If TSH is suppressed but fT4 is normal, measure free T3 (fT3).
- For patients with overt Graves' hyperthyroidism, treatment options include antithyroid drugs (ATDs), radioiodine (RAI) therapy, or thyroidectomy.
- If ATDs are selected as the primary treatment for Graves' disease (GD), continue the medication for 12 to 18 months, then discontinue if TSH levels normalize.
- If surgery is chosen as the primary treatment for GD, near-total or total thyroidectomy is

preferred and should be performed by a high-volume thyroid surgeon.

- For patients with overt toxic multinodular goiter (TMNG) or toxic adenoma (TA), consider RAI therapy or thyroidectomy. Long-term, low-dose methimazole (MMI) may be appropriate in certain cases.

- During febrile illnesses or at the onset of pharyngitis, obtain a differential white blood cell count for all patients on antithyroid medications.

- Assess liver function and hepatocellular integrity in patients taking MMI or propylthiouracil (PTU) who exhibit symptoms such as pruritic rash, jaundice, light-colored stools, dark urine, joint pain, abdominal pain, bloating, anorexia, nausea, or fatigue.

- Levothyroxine is the preferred treatment for hypothyroidism. The main therapeutic goals are:

  i) Resolution of symptoms and improvement in biological and physiological markers of hypothyroidism.

  ii) Normalization of serum TSH levels and improvement in thyroid hormone concentrations.

iii) Prevention of iatrogenic thyrotoxicosis or overtreatment, especially in the elderly.

- To enhance absorption, levothyroxine should be taken on an empty stomach, either 1 hour before breakfast or at bedtime, at least 3 hours after the last meal. However, consistent daily intake before breakfast may improve patient adherence.

Levothyroxine Replacement Therapy

Levothyroxine replacement can be initiated either as a full or partial replacement therapy, with gradual dose adjustments based on serum TSH levels. Adjustments should be made in response to significant changes in body weight, pregnancy, or aging. Serum TSH levels should be re-evaluated 4 to 8 weeks following any dose modification.

Subclinical Thyroid Disorders

- For individuals over 65 years of age with persistently low TSH (<0.1 mIU/L), treatment

for subclinical hyperthyroidism (SCHyper) is recommended.
- Antithyroid drugs should be the initial treatment choice for subclinical hyperthyroidism, regardless of its cause.
- In cases of persistent or worsening subclinical hyperthyroidism due to autonomous nodules or multinodular goiter, radioactive iodine therapy should be considered.
- To diagnose subclinical hypothyroidism, elevated TSH levels should be confirmed with repeated measurements.

Thyroid Nodules/Goiter

- Patients with suspected thyroid nodules or nodular goiter, or incidental findings of thyroid abnormalities on imaging, should undergo a dedicated thyroid and neck ultrasound that includes both the thyroid and surrounding neck compartments.
- Surgery is indicated in the following situations:
  i. Symptomatic compression or large goiters (>80 g).

ii. Low radioactive iodine uptake.

iii. Documented or suspected thyroid malignancy (e.g., suspicious or indeterminate cytology).

iv. Large thyroid nodules, particularly those larger than 4 cm or those that are non functioning or hypofunctioning on 123I or 99mTc pertechnetate scans.

v. Coexisting hyperparathyroidism requiring surgical intervention.

vi. High levels of TRAb.

vii. Moderate-to-severe active Graves' ophthalmopathy (GO).

- Surgery is generally not recommended for patients with significant comorbidities such as severe cardiopulmonary disease, end-stage cancer, or other debilitating conditions, or in cases where access to a high-volume thyroid surgeon is limited.
- Subacute thyroiditis should be considered in patients presenting with a painful goiter.

Thyroid Storm

- The diagnosis of thyroid storm is primarily clinical. While both the BWPS and JTA diagnostic tools can assist in diagnosis, the BWPS is preferred due to its higher sensitivity.
- For thyroid storms, administer high doses of propylthiouracil (PTU) initially (500–1000 mg loading dose, followed by 250 mg every 4–6 hours). If PTU is contraindicated, high doses of methimazole (MMI) (60–80 mg/day) can be used as an alternative.
- Beta-adrenergic blockers, such as propranolol, should be used to manage heart rate and mitigate the peripheral effects of excess thyroid hormone.
- In cases where beta-adrenergic blockers are contraindicated, shorter-acting intravenous options such as esmolol or diltiazem can be employed to control heart rate.
- Administer high doses of glucocorticoids (e.g., intravenous hydrocortisone 100 mg every 6 hours or dexamethasone 2 mg every 6 hours) during a thyroid storm.
- Provide 5–10 drops of Lugol's iodine every 6–8 hours for the first 10 days, following the

administration of antithyroid drugs, to rapidly improve thyrotoxicosis.

- Patients with thyroid storms should receive early definitive treatment with radioactive iodine (RAI). For those with large obstructing goiters or contraindications to RAI, early thyroidectomy should be considered.

Myxedema Coma

- Begin with intravenous hydrocortisone (200 mg initially, then 100 mg every 6–8 hours) before administering levothyroxine.
- Follow with an initial intravenous dose of levothyroxine (200–400 mcg), then continue with 1.6 mcg/kg/day (75% of the oral dose) if administered intravenously. If intravenous levothyroxine is unavailable, administer oral levothyroxine as a 500 mcg loading dose followed by a maintenance dose.
- Intravenous liothyronine may be used in addition to levothyroxine if available, with a loading dose of 5–20 mcg followed by 2.5–10

mcg every 8 hours until the patient regains consciousness.

Pre-/Perioperative Management

- Elective surgeries should be deferred until the patient achieves euthyroidism or a near-euthyroid state.
- For hyperthyroid patients requiring urgent surgery, rapidly control the condition with high doses of MMI or PTU, beta-blockers, Lugol's iodine, and glucocorticoids.

Thyroid Disorders in Pregnancy

- Pregnant women with overt hypothyroidism should be treated with levothyroxine (LT4).
- For maternal subclinical hypothyroidism, LT4 treatment is recommended to minimize the risk of miscarriage and preterm delivery in the following cases:
    a) In pregnant women with negative TPO antibodies:

- LT4 is advised if TSH levels exceed 10 mIU/L.

   - LT4 may be considered if TSH is above the pregnancy-specific reference range or 4.0 mIU/L.

  b) In pregnant women with positive TPO antibodies:

   - LT4 is recommended if TSH is above the pregnancy-specific reference range or 4.0 mIU/L.

   - LT4 may be considered if TSH is greater than 2.5 mIU/L.

- For women who were on LT4 prior to conception, the target TSH level should be no higher than 2.5 mIU/L before conception and during the first trimester.

- During the second and third trimesters, the target TSH level can be set at 3.0 mIU/L or lower.

- Pregnant women who were on LT4 before conception should have their LT4 dosage increased by 30%–50% upon conception, with the higher end of the range for post-ablative hypothyroidism and the lower end for autoimmune hypothyroidism.

- If a suppressed TSH and elevated free T4 are observed in the first trimester, a clinical history and physical examination are needed to determine the cause. Graves' disease should be differentiated from gestational thyrotoxicosis clinically, with TRAb supporting the diagnosis of Graves' disease.

- Gestational transient thyrotoxicosis is primarily managed with supportive measures: rehydration and hospitalization if hyperemesis gravidarum is present, and beta-blockers if symptoms are severe. Antithyroid drugs are not recommended.

- If antithyroid drugs are necessary during pregnancy, propylthiouracil (PTU) is recommended for use throughout the first trimester.

- Use the lowest effective dose of antithyroid drugs to manage thyrotoxicosis during pregnancy, aiming to keep free T4 within or moderately above the reference range.

- For postpartum thyroiditis:

- Women in the thyrotoxic phase who are symptomatic should be treated with beta-blockers; antithyroid drugs are not recommended.

- Women in the hypothyroid phase who are symptomatic should receive thyroxine. Those with mild symptoms who choose not to be treated should have their thyroid function tests monitored every 4–8 weeks until euthyroidism is achieved.

Adolescents

-Hypothyroidism Due to Hashimoto's Thyroiditis: Levothyroxine is the recommended treatment, with dosage based on body weight or body surface area. The target range for TSH should be in the lower half of the reference range, while free T4 should be in the upper half. Levothyroxine can effectively reduce thyroid gland size or goiter.

-Non-Goitrous Euthyroid Hashimoto's Thyroiditis: Monitor for goiter, antithyroid antibodies, and thyroid function patterns. Treatment with thyroxine in these cases remains debated.

-Hyperthyroidism: The initial treatment of choice is antithyroid drugs (ATDs), such as carbimazole or its active form, methimazole (MMI). The usual dose is 0.2–0.5 mg/kg daily, with a maximum initial dose of 30 mg per day. After 2–4 weeks, once thyroid hormone levels normalize, the dose should be reduced by 30%–50%. TSH levels, which may take 2–4 months to stabilize, should not be used to adjust the dosage. If serious adverse reactions to MMI occur, consider radioactive iodine (RAI) or surgery, as PTU carries higher risks than RAI or surgery.

-Hyperthyroidism: Avoid using propylthiouracil (PTU) in children. If PTU is used, discontinue it immediately and assess liver function if the child shows symptoms such as anorexia, pruritus, rash, jaundice, light-colored stool, dark urine, joint pain, abdominal pain, or malaise, due to the risk of severe liver complications.

-Hyperthyroidism: Definitive treatments for Graves' disease include RAI or thyroidectomy. Consider definitive therapy for children if there is relapse after adequate ATD treatment, non-compliance, or adverse effects from ATDs. The duration of ATD therapy before considering RAI or surgery remains a topic of debate.

Thyroid Disorders in the Elderly

Subclinical Hypothyroidism:
  - For patients over 70 years old, consider levothyroxine treatment if serum TSH is ≥10 mIU/L and symptoms of hypothyroidism or high vascular risk are present.
  - For patients over 70 years old, if serum TSH is ≤10 mIU/L, monitor and repeat thyroid function tests in 6 months.
  - For patients 70 years old or younger, consider levothyroxine treatment if serum TSH is ≥10 mIU/L.

- For patients 70 years old or younger with serum TSH ≤10 mIU/L and symptoms of hypothyroidism, consider a 3-month trial of levothyroxine, followed by an assessment of treatment response.

For Patients Aged ≤70 Years:

- If serum TSH is ≤10 mIU/L and there are no symptoms of hypothyroidism, observe the patient and repeat thyroid function tests in 6 months.

Drug-Induced Thyroid Disorders:

- Monitor thyroid function tests before starting amiodarone, then 3–4 months after initiation, and at 3–6 month intervals thereafter. Continue monitoring for up to 1 year after discontinuing amiodarone.

Graves' Ophthalmopathy:

- Assess Graves' ophthalmopathy (GO) by evaluating both activity and severity using standardized criteria. GO can be classified as active or inactive, and further categorized as mild, moderate, severe, or sight-threatening.
- Restore euthyroidism as promptly as possible in patients with GO.
- For patients with mild-to-moderate GO undergoing radioiodine therapy, a prophylactic oral prednisolone regimen of 0.4 -- 0.5 mg/kg/day for 3 months is recommended.

Levels of Evidence:

- Level I: Evidence from at least one well-conducted randomized controlled trial.
- Level II-1: Evidence from well-designed controlled trials without randomization.
- Level II-2: Evidence from well-designed cohort or case-control studies, preferably from multiple centers or groups.
- Level II-3: Evidence from multiple time series with or without intervention, or dramatic results

from uncontrolled experiments (e.g., early penicillin treatment results).

- Level III: Opinions of respected authorities based on clinical experience, descriptive studies, case reports, or expert committee reports.

Glossary

Antithyroid Drugs (ATDs)
Medications used to reduce thyroid hormone production in hyperthyroidism, including methimazole and propylthiouracil.

Calcitonin
A hormone produced by the thyroid gland that helps regulate calcium levels in the blood.

Dysthyroid Optic Neuropathy (DON)
A severe form of Graves' ophthalmopathy characterized by compression of the optic nerve, leading to vision impairment.

Euthyroid
A state in which thyroid hormone levels are normal and the thyroid gland is functioning properly.

Fine Needle Aspiration Biopsy (FNAB)

A minimally invasive procedure used to extract cells from a thyroid nodule or goiter for diagnostic examination.

Graves' Ophthalmopathy (GO)
An autoimmune condition associated with hyperthyroidism, characterized by inflammation and swelling of the tissues around the eyes.

Hyperthyroidism
A condition where the thyroid gland is overactive and produces excessive thyroid hormones, leading to an increased metabolic rate.

Hypothyroidism
A condition where the thyroid gland is underactive and does not produce enough thyroid hormones, resulting in a decreased metabolic rate.

Methylprednisolone
A type of corticosteroid medication used to reduce inflammation, often used in high doses to

treat moderate-to-severe Graves' ophthalmopathy.

Radioactive Iodine (RAI) Therapy
A treatment for hyperthyroidism and thyroid cancer that uses radioactive iodine to destroy overactive thyroid cells.

Thyroid Scintigraphy
A diagnostic imaging technique that uses radioactive tracers to evaluate thyroid gland function and structure.

Thyroid Stimulating Hormone (TSH)
A hormone produced by the pituitary gland that stimulates the thyroid gland to produce thyroid hormones.

Thyroidectomy
Surgical removal of all or part of the thyroid gland, often performed to treat thyroid cancer or severe hyperthyroidism.

Thyroxine (T4)

One of the primary hormones produced by the thyroid gland, important for regulating metabolism and energy levels.

Triiodothyronine (T3)
A thyroid hormone that plays a critical role in regulating metabolism, heart rate, and body temperature.

Thyroid Autoantibodies
Antibodies produced by the immune system that target thyroid gland tissues, commonly seen in autoimmune thyroid diseases such as Graves' disease and Hashimoto's thyroiditis.

Thyroid Storm
A life-threatening condition characterized by an extreme exacerbation of hyperthyroidism symptoms, requiring immediate medical attention.

Thyroid Nodules

Lumps or growths in the thyroid gland, which can be benign or malignant and may require evaluation through imaging and biopsy.

Thyroiditis
Inflammation of the thyroid gland, which can be caused by various factors including autoimmune diseases, infections, or medications.

References

1. Shahar MA, Omar AM, Ab Wahab N, et al. (for the MyENDO Study Group). The prevalence of overt and subclinical thyroid disorders in Malaysia's adult population. Int J Thyroidol. 2017;10(Suppl 1):S177.

2. Shahar MA, Omar AM, Ab Wahab N, et al. (for the MyENDO Study Group). Increased prevalence of goiter but not thyroid nodules among younger age groups in Malaysia. Proc 12th Asia Ocean Thyroid Assoc Congr. Int J Thyroidol. 2017;10(Suppl 1):S128.

3. Shahar MA, Omar AM, Ab Wahab N, et al. (for the MyENDO Study Group). Elevated thyroid antibody levels in urban and coastal populations of Malaysia. Proc 12th Asia Ocean Thyroid Assoc Congr. Int J Thyroidol. 2017;10(Suppl 1):S209.

4. Ross DS, Burch HB, Cooper DS, et al. 2016 American Thyroid Association guidelines for the diagnosis and management of hyperthyroidism and other causes of thyrotoxicosis. Thyroid. 2016;26(10):1343–1421.

5. Williams I, Ankrett VO, Lazarus JH, et al. Causes of hyperthyroidism in Canada and Wales. J Epidemiol Community Health. 1983;37(3):245–248.

6. Ahsan T, Banu Z, Jabeen R, et al. Clinical spectrum and various forms of thyrotoxicosis at the endocrine clinic of Jinnah Postgraduate Medical Centre. J Pak Med Assoc. 2013;63(3):354–357.

7. Brix TH, Hansen PS, Hegedus L, et al. Revisiting Yersinia infection in the etiology of Graves' disease: Evidence from a twin case-control study. Clin Endocrinol (Oxf). 2008;69(3):491–496.

9. Mirfakhraee S, Mathews D, Peng L, et al. A solitary hyperfunctioning thyroid nodule with thyroid carcinoma: A literature review. Thyroid Res. 2013;6(1):7.

10. Jaeschke H, Schaarschmidt J, Eszlinger M, et al. Identification of a new TSHR variant (L665F) associated with non-autoimmune hyperthyroidism. J Clin Endocrinol Metab. 2014;99(10):E2051–E2059.

11. Raman L, Murray J, Banka R. Primary tuberculosis of the thyroid gland: An unexpected cause of thyrotoxicosis. BMJ Case Rep. 2014. doi:10.1136/bcr-2013-202792.

12. Puri MM, Dougall P, Arora VK. Tuberculosis of the thyroid gland. Med J Malaysia. 2002;57(2):237–239.

13. Yahaya N, Din SW, Ghazali MZ, et al. Primary thyroid lymphoma with elevated free thyroxine levels. Singapore Med J. 2011;52(9):e173–176.

14. Merza Z, White D, Khanem N. Struma during pregnancy: An uncommon cause of hyperthyroidism. Clin Nucl Med. 2015;40(8):687–688.

15. Gardner D, Ho SC. Functioning thyroid metastases as a rare cause of hyperthyroidism. BMJ Case Rep. 2014. doi:10.1136/bcr-2014-206468.

16. Hoang TD, Mai VQ, Clyde PW, et al. Over-the-counter drug-induced thyroid disorders. Endocr Pract. 2013;19(2):268–274.

17. Dimeski G, Lampe G, Brown NN. Thyrotoxicosis due to Chinese herbal supplements. Pathology. 2013;45(2):185–186.

18. Wartique L, Pothen LA, Prison N, et al. An unusual cause of epidemic thyrotoxicosis. Acta Clin Belg. 2017;72(6):451–453.

19. Marchand L, Chabert P, Chaudesaygues E, et al. An unusual cause of cardiothyreosis. Gynaecol Endocrinol. 2016;32(2):107–109.

20. Foppiani L, Cascio C, Lo Pinto G. Iodine-induced hyperthyroidism as a combination of different etiologies: An overlooked entity in the elderly. Aging Clin Exp Res. 2016;28(5):1023–1027.

21. Dave A, Ludlow J, Malaty J. Thyrotoxicosis: An under-recognized etiology. BMJ Case Rep. 2015. doi:10.1136/bcr-2014-208119.

22. Fricke E, Fricke H, Esdom E, et al. Scintigraphy for risk assessment of iodine-induced thyrotoxicosis in patients receiving contrast agents for coronary angiography: A prospective study. J Clin Endocrinol Metab. 2004;89(12):6092–6096.

23. Van der Molen AJ, Thomsen HS, Morcos SK. Impact of iodinated contrast media on

thyroid function in adults. Eur Radiol. 2004;14(5):902–907.

24. Tsang W, Houlden RL. Amiodarone-induced thyrotoxicosis: A review. Can J Cardiol. 2009;25(7):421–424

25. KF Lee, Lee KM, Fung TT. Amiodarone-induced thyroid dysfunction in the Chinese population of Hong Kong. Hong Kong Med J. 2010;16(6):434–439.

26. Zosin I, Balas M, et al. Amiodarone-induced thyroid dysfunction in areas with sufficient iodine: Epidemiological and clinical data. Polish J Endocrinol. 2012;63(1):2–9.

27. Fadilah SA, Faridah I, Cheong SK. Transient hyperthyroidism following L-asparaginase treatment for acute lymphoblastic leukemia. Med J Malaysia. 2000;55(4):513–515.

28. AVS AK, Mohan A, Kumar PG, et al. Scintigraphic profiles of patients with thyrotoxicosis and their correlation with biochemical and sonological findings. J Clin Diagn Res. 2017;11(5):OC01–OC03.

29. Alzahrani AS, Ceresini G, Aldasouqi SA. The role of ultrasonography in differentiating thyrotoxicosis: A noninvasive, cost-effective, yet underutilized diagnostic tool. Endocr Pract. 2012;18(4):567–578.

30. Bartalena L. Global overview of the diagnosis and management of Graves' disease. Nat Rev Endocrinol. 2013;9:724–734.

31. Bartalena L, Burch HB, Burman KD, et al. A 2013 European survey of clinical practice patterns for managing Graves' disease. Clin Endocrinol (Oxf). 2016;84(1):115–120.

32. Hesaraghatta SA, Abraham P. Utilizing TSH receptor antibody measurements to guide

treatment decisions in Graves' disease. Clin Endocrinol (Oxf). 2017;86(5):652–657.

33. Kahaly GJ, Olivo PD. Graves' disease. N Engl J Med. 2017;376:184.

34. Kahaly GJ, Diana T. Functionality and nomenclature of TSH receptor antibodies. Front Endocrinol (Lausanne). 2017;8:28.

35. Schott M, Hermsen D, Broecker-Preuss M, et al. Clinical efficacy of the first automated TSH receptor autoantibodies assay for diagnosing Graves' disease: An international multicenter trial. Clin Endocrinol (Oxf). 2009;71(4):566–573.

36. Diana T, Wuster C, Kanitz M, et al. Variable sensitivity of five binding assays and two bioassays for TSH receptor antibodies. J Endocrinol Invest. 2016;39(10):1159–1165.

37. Diana T, Wüster C, Olivo PD, et al. Performance and specificity of six

immunoassays for TSH receptor antibodies: A multicenter evaluation. Eur Thyroid J. 2017;6(5):243–249.

38. Kotwal A, Stan M. Overview of thyrotropin receptor antibodies. Ophthalmic Plast Reconstr Surg. 2018;34(4S Suppl 1):S20–S27.

39. Sipos JA, Kahaly GJ. Imaging techniques for thyrotoxicosis. Am J Med. 2012;125(9):S1–S2.

40. Meller J, Becker W. The continued relevance of thyroid scintigraphy in the era of advanced ultrasound technology. Eur J Nucl Med. 2002;Suppl 2:S425–S438.

41. Bahn Chair RS, Burch HB, Cooper DS, et al. Management guidelines for hyperthyroidism and other causes of thyrotoxicosis by the American Thyroid Association and the American Association of Clinical Endocrinologists. Thyroid. 2011;21(6):593–646.

42. Biondi B, Cooper DS. Clinical significance of subclinical thyroid dysfunction. Endocr Rev. 2008;29(1):76–131.

43. Madariaga GA, Palacios SS, Guillen-Grima F, et al. Incidence and prevalence of thyroid dysfunction in Europe: A meta-analysis. J Clin Endocrinol Metab. 2014;99(3):923–931.

44. Biondi B, Bartalena L, Cooper DS, et al. 2015 European Thyroid Association guidelines for diagnosing and treating endogenous subclinical hyperthyroidism. Eur Thyroid J. 2015;4(3):149–163.

45. Lim KK, Wong M, Mohamud WN, et al. Effects of iodized salt supplementation on thyroid status among the Orang Asli in Hulu Selangor, Malaysia. Asia Pac J Clin Nutr. 2013;22(1):41–47.

46. Chin KY, Ima-Nirwana S, Mohamed IN, et al. Association of thyroid-stimulating hormone

levels with bone health status in men. Int J Med Sci. 2013;10(7):857–863.

47. Mai VQ, Burch HB. A structured approach to evaluating and treating subclinical hyperthyroidism. Endocr Pract. 2012;18(5):772–780.

48. Abdul Shakoor SA, Hawkins R, Kua SY, et al. Natural history and comorbidities in subjects with subclinical hyperthyroidism: Insights from a tertiary hospital setting. Ann Acad Med Singapore. 2014;43:506–510.

49. Schouten BJ, Brownlie BE, Frampton CM, et al. Predictors of outcomes in subclinical thyrotoxicosis in an outpatient setting. Clin Endocrinol (Oxf). 2011;74(2):257–261.

50. Asvold BO, Bjoro T, Nilsen TI, et al. Thyrotropin levels and risk of fatal coronary heart disease: Results from the HUNT study. Arch Intern Med. 2008;168(8):855–860.

51. Collet TH, Gussekloo J, Bauer DC, et al. explored the association between subclinical hyperthyroidism and the increased likelihood of coronary heart disease and mortality in their study. Archives of Internal Medicine, 2012;172(10):799-809.

52. Sawin CT, Geller A, Wolf PA, et al. identified a correlation between low serum thyrotropin levels and heightened atrial fibrillation risk in older adults. New England Journal of Medicine, 1994;331:1249-1252.

53. Rodondi N, Newman AB, Vittinghoff E, et al. investigated subclinical hypothyroidism's connection to heart failure, cardiovascular events, and mortality. Archives of Internal Medicine, 2005;65(21):2460-2466.

54. Yang LB, Jiang DQ, Qi WB, et al. conducted a meta-analysis on subclinical hyperthyroidism's influence on cardiovascular events and all-cause

mortality. European Journal of Endocrinology, 2012;167(1):75-84.

55. Walsh JP, Bremner AP, Bulsara AK, et al. studied the relationship between subclinical thyroid dysfunction and cardiovascular disease risk. Archives of Internal Medicine, 2005;165(21):2467-2472.

56. Yang R, Yao L, Fang Y, et al. explored the link between subclinical thyroid dysfunction and fracture risk or low bone mineral density through a systematic review and meta-analysis. Journal of Bone and Mineral Metabolism, 2018;36(2):209-220.

57. Garin MC, Arnold AM, Lee JS, et al. assessed subclinical thyroid dysfunction's influence on hip fracture and bone mineral density among older adults. Journal of Clinical Endocrinology & Metabolism, 2014;99(8):2657-2664.

58. Cappola AR, Fried LP, Arnold AM, et al. examined the interplay between thyroid status, cardiovascular risk, and mortality in an aging population. JAMA, 2006;295(9):1033-1041.

59. Chaker L, Baumgartner C, Ikram MA, et al. performed a systematic review and meta-analysis on subclinical thyroid dysfunction and its risk of stroke. European Journal of Epidemiology, 2014;29(11):791-800.

60. Formiga F, FerrarA, Padros G, et al. analyzed thyroid status and its relation to functional, cognitive status, and survival over a three-year follow-up period in the OCTABAIX study. European Journal of Endocrinology, 2013;170(1):69-75.

61. Rieben C, Segna D, da Costa BR, et al. conducted a meta-analysis on subclinical thyroid dysfunction and its potential to contribute to cognitive decline, drawing from prospective cohort studies. Journal of Clinical

Endocrinology & Metabolism, 2016;101(12):4945-4954.

62. Stott DJ, McLellan AR, Finlayson J, et al. discovered that elderly patients with suppressed TSH but normal thyroid hormone levels often experience mild thyroid overactivity and increased risk of overt hyperthyroidism. QJM, 1991;78(285):77-84.

63. Sgarbi JA, Villaca FG, Garbeline B, et al. investigated the benefits of early antithyroid treatment on clinical and cardiac abnormalities in subclinical hyperthyroidism. Journal of Clinical Endocrinology & Metabolism, 2003;88(4):1672-1677.

64. Faber J, Jensen IW, Petersen L, et al. examined the effects of radioiodine treatment on bone loss in postmenopausal women with subclinical hyperthyroidism. Clinical Endocrinology (Oxford), 1998;48(3):285-290.

65. Greenlund LJ, Nair KS, Brennan MD, et al. documented changes in body composition in women following treatment for overt and subclinical hyperthyroidism. Endocrine Practice, 2008;14(8):973-978.

66. Nacar AB, Acar G, Yorgun H, et al. examined how antithyroid treatment affects atrial conduction times in patients with subclinical hyperthyroidism. Echocardiography, 2012;29(8):950-955.

67. Biondi B, Fazio S, Carella C, et al. demonstrated that beta-blockade effectively controls adrenergic overactivity, improving the quality of life in patients on long-term suppressive levothyroxine therapy. Journal of Clinical Endocrinology & Metabolism, 1994;78(5):1028-1033.

68. Bolk N, Visser TJ, Nijman J, et al. conducted a randomized double-blind crossover trial to compare the effects of evening versus morning

levothyroxine intake. Archives of Internal Medicine, 2010;170(22):1996-2002.

We Appreciate Your Feedback!

Thank you for choosing *COMPREHENSIVE GUIDELINES FOR THYROID DISORDER MANAGEMENT: Innovative Approaches for Optimal Patient Outcomes*. We hope this book has been a valuable resource in your understanding and management of thyroid disorders.

If you found the content useful, we would be grateful if you could take a moment to share your honest thoughts by leaving a review on Amazon KDP. Your feedback helps us improve and assists other readers in finding the resources they need.

To leave a review, visit our Amazon KDP page and share your experience. We truly appreciate your time and support.

Thank you once again for your engagement!

Warm regards,

Dr. Yoshiki Kiyomizu
Clinical Researcher, Keio University Hospital, Tokyo, Japan

www.ingramcontent.com/pod-product-compliance
Lightning Source LLC
Chambersburg PA
CBHW052138220526
45471CB00004B/1437